ALTERNATIVE
BIRTH
The Complete Guide

ALTERNATIVE BIRTH

The Complete Guide

Healthy Options for You and Your Baby

CARL JONES

Foreword by
Dr. Celeste R. Phillips

Introduction by
Donald Creevy, M.D.

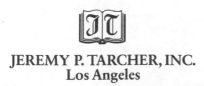

JEREMY P. TARCHER, INC.
Los Angeles

Photographs for chapters one, three, five, seven, and the Epilogue were taken by Noa Ben-Amotz. Photographs for the Introduction, chapters two, four, and six were taken by Byron F. Greatorex. The photograph for chapter eight was taken by Dr. Michael J. Rosenthal, Medical Director of the Family Birthing Center of Upland, California.

Library of Congress Cataloging in Publication Data

Jones, Carl.
    Alternative birth, the complete guide: healthy options for you and your baby / Carl Jones ; foreword by Celeste Phillips ; introduction by Donald Creevy.—1st ed.
    p. cm.
ISBN 0-87477-616-3
    1. Natural childbirth.   I. Title.
RG661.J577   1990
618.4 ' 5—dc20

Jeremy P. Tarcher, Inc.
5858 Wilshire Blvd., Suite 200
Los Angeles, CA 90036

Distributed by St. Martin's Press, New York

Design by Lee Fukui

Manufactured in the United States of America
10 9 8 7 6 5 4 3 2 1
First Edition

Contents

To Eric

Acknowledgments

THANK YOU TO EVERYONE WHO helped me complete this book. Dozens of childbirth professionals read portions of this book and made numerous suggestions, improving it.

Those who contributed ideas to the chapter "Midwifery Care" include Joan Remington, of the Arizona School of Midwifery; Jo Anne Myers-Ciecko, of the Seattle Midwifery School; Lorri Walker, CNM of Southern California; Quila Rider, CNM of Southern California; Alice Bailes, CNM of Virginia; and Laurie Foster, a Vermont midwife.

My wife, Jan, and I both thank Barbara Mason for inviting us to a birth at the wonderful Marchbanks Alternative Birthing Center in La Habra, California. This was the first birth—other than her own—that my wife had attended.

People who contributed ideas to the chapter "Birth in a Child-bearing Center" include Barbara Mason, of the Marchbanks Alternative Birthing Center in La Habra, California; Ruth Watson Lubic, of the Maternity Center Association in New York; Karen Knudson, of BirthPlace in Pittsburgh, Pennsylvania; Mary Hammond-Tooke, of the Maternity Center in Baltimore, Maryland; Vicky Wolfrum, of South Bay Family Care in San Pedro, California; and CharLynn Doughtry, of the Labor of Love Childbirth Center in Lakeland, Florida.

Those who contributed suggestions to the "Waterbirth" chapter include Susanna Napierala, midwife of Glen Ellen, California, and Barbara Harper, of Waterbirth International in Santa Barbara, California.

People who contributed suggestions to the chapter about birth in the hospital include Celeste Phillips, Clinical Obstetrical Specialist in the Surgeon General's Office; Colleen Gerlach, of Birth Place at Riverside Medical Center in Minneapolis; and many other nurses, midwives, and physicians.

My special thanks to Anne Cleary Sommers, editor of *MOM* magazine, who encouraged me throughout this project and who spent many hours driving me to childbirth professionals and birth centers when I was conducting workshops in Southern California.

I am particularly indebted to the hundreds of parents throughout the United States who have shared their birth experiences with me. This has helped me to learn about childbirth in a wide variety of circumstances.

Thanks also to Andrea Stein, my editor, to Jennifer Boynton and Paul Murphy in production, and the rest of the good folk at Jeremy Tarcher, including the always-pleasant receptionist. All have been very patient and helpful.

Preface

THIS IS A BOOK ABOUT CHOICE. The material presented in this book can help you make a decision about the most appropriate place of birth for you and your child.

For most people, childbirth is wellness, not illness. In addition to the birth of a baby, childbirth represents the beginning of a family. Thus, birth is a very important event in people's lives and deserves thoughtful consideration about the place in which it will occur.

Today the childbearing woman has many options. To choose the right health-care provider and birthing place for yourself and your family will not be easy. That decision-making process can be helped by the information provided in this book. Carl Jones describes today's options and presents advantages and disadvantages for you to consider. Read it and talk about the birth options he presents with your partner, family, and health care provider. Ask questions about any of the information in this book that you want to know more about, and get the answers before making your decision about the place of birth for your baby.

Your birth is just that . . . yours. It is a special time in your life that you may choose to keep for yourself and your partner or share with others you love. Whatever that decision is, it is *yours*. Become informed about your options, make safe and appropriate choices, and the birth of your baby will be the happiest day of your life.

Dr. Celeste R. Phillips
Clinical Obstetrical Specialist,
The Surgeon-General's Office

Foreword

WHERE WILL YOU GIVE BIRTH? At home, in a birth center, or in a hospital? On the birthing bed, on the floor, or in a tub of warm water? Who will attend the birth: a midwife, family physician, or obstetrician? What medical interventions are appropriate? Which are safe for you and your baby?

This is a book about choices in childbirth. It is written for all who have an interest in pregnancy and birth—expectant mothers, expectant fathers, siblings-to-be, childbirth educators, midwives, physicians, childbirth assistants, and administrators.

As Leboyer has given us a new approach to childbirth in his concept of gentle birth, Carl Jones has given us a new model of labor with his *laboring mind response*. The *laboring mind response*— a clear description of how the body and mind interact during childbirth—is a breakthrough. It will enable you to understand why guided imagery is such a powerful way to reduce the fear and pain of labor. And it will show you why the childbirth alternatives discussed in this book are almost always more satisfying than traditional hospital birth.

The underlying theme of this book is the inalienable right of parents to choose where, when, how, and with whom they give birth.

Carl Jones never hides his own point of view on any aspect of pregnancy and birth. You always know where he stands: he is the mother's advocate. At the same time, he never fails to present a balanced discussion of alternatives. He provides the tools you need to make choices for yourself.

Everyone from the novice lay midwife to the experienced perinatologist agrees that the safety of mother and baby is of the utmost importance in every birth. However, there is widespread disagreement about what constitutes safety in birth, and about how the mother can maximize her chance of the safest birth. Carl Jones discusses the alternatives open to each mother and documents his discussion with references from medical literature.

Once you have read this book, you will be equipped to make rational, informed choices for yourself. You will be confident in the knowledge that you have explored each choice to the fullest. You will be well prepared to plan the birth that best suits your own personal needs and desires. And most importantly, you will know how to choose the care provider and place of birth that is best for you.

Dr. Donald Creevy
Clinical Assistant Professor
of Obstetrics and Gynecology,
Stanford University School of Medicine

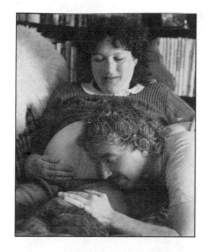

Giving Birth Your Way

GIVING BIRTH CAN BE ONE OF the most beautiful and memorable events in your life. The birth of a baby is one of nature's most awesome miracles, and few things elicit such profound emotions—joy, elation, and love. Nothing compares to reaching down and receiving your own child as he or she enters the world wriggling with life.

Every labor, like every person, is unique, and all parents have somewhat different goals and expectations about their birth experience. However, all want a healthy baby, a safe birth, and a positive experience. They deserve to enjoy this adventure to the fullest, and every child deserves to be born into a loving setting.

Fulfilling these goals is what this book is about. It is the reason hundreds of thousands of parents throughout the world choose one of the alternative-birth options described in the chapters ahead.

This book will acquaint you with a number of choices for a healthy, rewarding birth so you can choose the method that is best for you and your baby. It will also provide all the information you need to shape your birth plans to your individual needs.

WHAT IS ALTERNATIVE BIRTH?

Alternative birth can be roughly defined as any childbirth method other than conventional hospital labor and delivery. In this book, I use the term *alternative birth* to include the following.

- midwife-attended birth in a home, a childbearing center, or a hospital (discussed in Chapter Four)
- birth at home (discussed in Chapter Five)
- birth in a childbearing center (discussed in Chapter Six)
- birth in a homelike setting within a hospital whose staff practices noninterventive maternity care (discussed in Chapter Seven)
- waterbirth, which can take place at home, in a childbearing center, and in a few hospitals (discussed in Chapter Eight).

Alternative birth encompasses a wide variety of options throughout the world. For example, in the United States home birth is considered an alternative, while in the Netherlands it is the norm. Likewise, some Americans think of a delivery attended by a midwife as an alternative birth. However, in Japan, which has the lowest infant-mortality rate in the world, midwives attend nearly all births. Dr. Marsden G. Wagner, the European Director of the World Health Organization, says that, "Every single country in the European Region with perinatal and infant-mortality rates lower than the United States uses midwives as the principal and only birth attendant for at least 70 percent of all births."

Some childbirth professionals as well as parents who have experienced an alternative birth do not like the term because *alternative* sometimes has a negative connotation. It may elicit images of a radical departure from conventional lifestyle—like living without electricity—or of being outside the mainstream. For many, this implies that alternatives are less valid or less acceptable. It is my hope, however, that the options discussed in this book will soon become the *mainstream,* and that such negative connotations may be eliminated altogether, for, as you will discover in the chapters ahead, these options are more rewarding, more satisfying, more humanizing, and safer than conventional hospital childbirth in almost every way.

Characteristics of Alternative Birth

Whether it takes place at home, in a childbearing center, or in a hospital, alternative birth is characterized by the following qualities.

- a philosophy of childbirth in which labor and birth are viewed as a natural and normal process, rather than as an illness or a clinical procedure

- a noninterventive approach to maternity care
- an active participation of the mother in her health care in which she, not her health-care providers, makes all major decisions
- an active participation of the mother, the father, and the entire family throughout the childbearing process
- a recognition that the baby is a conscious participant in the birth process who deserves the most gentle and least traumatic beginning to life outside the womb

WHY CHOOSE AN ALTERNATIVE BIRTH?

A revolution in the way women give birth is taking place throughout the world. Alternative birth is part of a major health-care trend in which more people are taking an active role in their health care. Increasing numbers are paying greater attention to nutrition, eating more whole foods, and turning to holistic health-care methods such as chiropractic care, herbal medicine, acupuncture, guided imagery, and other forms of healing—all of which are considered alternatives to conventional medicine.

However, a number of other factors have contributed to the increasing popularity of alternative birth, including childbirth education, the women's movement, dissatisfaction with conventional hospital birth, a desire for more control of the childbearing process, and a need for more personalized maternity care.

Childbirth education probably has played the largest role in revolutionizing childbirth customs. One of the pioneers in this field was British physician Grantly Dick-Read, who in the 1940s presented convincing arguments against then-common obstetric practices such as leaving laboring women alone or giving them excessive amounts of medication. He stressed the importance of recognizing the psychological factors that influence childbearing. Dr. Dick-Read believed that the pain of labor was the direct result of the mother's fear and tension and that without this fear and tension, childbirth would be nearly painless. To decrease these negative responses, he advocated acquainting the mother with the normal process of birth through childbirth education. He also believed in providing emotional support with the presence of the father or another familiar person during labor. While few agree with Dr. Dick-Read's view that childbirth would be painless in the absence of fear and tension, his emphasis on these positive changes had enormous influence. His work contributed to the founding of the International Childbirth Education Association (ICEA), a group of childbirth educators. Formed in 1960, ICEA had nearly twelve thousand members in thirty-one countries by 1984.

Meanwhile, during the 1950s, Soviet physicians developed the *psychoprophylactic method* to control fear and pain during labor. This was based on educating pregnant women about the anatomy and physiology of childbearing and teaching them to respond to uterine contractions with patterned breathing and relaxation. This method was introduced to France by French physician Fernand Lamaze in 1958. An American woman, Marjorie Karmel, who gave birth in Dr. Lamaze's French clinic, founded the American Society for Psychoprophylaxis in Obstetrics (ASPO) in 1960 to teach the Lamaze method. By 1986 there were ten thousand Lamaze instructors (though their teaching has been modified several times over the years). The Lamaze method continues to be popular in both traditional hospital births and alternative births.

During the last couple of decades, some thirty thousand childbirth educators have been certified by ICEA, ASPO, and smaller childbirth-education organizations including Informed Homebirth (IH), The Academy of Certified Childbirth Educators (ACCE), The American Academy of Husband Coached Childbirth (AAHCC), and others. (For more information on these groups, see Resources.) Some childbirth educators teach more about alternative birth than others, but most have educated parents to become more active participants in their birthing, which has added to the tremendous expansion of awareness about labor and birth. The InterNational Association for Parents and Professionals for Safe Alternatives in Childbirth (NAPSAC) has contributed to the alternative-birth movement by disseminating information about the safety of home birth, midwifery care, and other nontraditional options.

The women's movement also has made a large contribution to an expansion of interest in alternative birth by making women aware of their rights in childbearing, and parents-to-be have started demanding more involvement in their own gynecologic and obstetric care.

Dissatisfaction with contemporary hospital birth began to grow as parents became aware that hospital birth had become a dehumanized event. A long list of hospital practices considered unnecessary and even inhumane includes separating mothers from their families; subjecting mothers to unpleasant, often unnecessary, and sometimes even hazardous procedures from the shaving of perineal hair to the overuse of medications; and separating babies and mothers after birth. Laboring women are frequently treated more like invalids with an illness rather than as the healthy women they are.

As their awareness has grown, parents have become fed up with the customs common in American hospitals and have sought alternatives. Every day parents are seeking alternatives, and one in four births is now considered to be an alternative birth. For example, one mother had her first child in a hospital where she had *epidural anesthesia* (numbing and immobilizing the body from the waist down) and an *episiotomy* (a surgical incision to widen the birth outlet) and where she gave birth with her legs in stirrups. She believed this was the way childbirth had to be. Later, she discovered that childbirth could be a much different experience; her next birth took place at home. "I loved staying at home," she says. "I didn't have to go anywhere during labor. I didn't have to submit my newborn to strangers. I didn't have to leave my other daughter for two to three days. I felt in control, as if I had really done everything myself."

In response to this dissatisfaction with traditional maternal care, hospitals have made tremendous improvements. In most, breastfeeding is now encouraged; and in many, birth is no longer a dehumanizing experience. In nearly all hospitals, fathers are welcome to attend labors and mothers and their newborns are not routinely separated. Yet physicians—not parents—still retain control of the events surrounding childbearing.

The parents' desire to control the events surrounding the childbearing process is another theme that has inspired the alternative-birth movement. Hundreds of thousands of parents have discovered that they have a right to decide how, when, and with whom they will give birth; in what position the mother will labor; how the father will take part in the childbearing process; and how they will address other concerns of maternity care. In addition, parents have become aware that the experience of childbirth, which is deeply meaningful, had lost its unique beauty—physically, psychologically, emotionally, and spiritually—in conventional hospitals.

In recent years many parents have chosen to give birth in places where their wishes come before policy, where the love bond between parent and child comes before obstetric protocol, where they can have personalized maternity care, and where they can be more comfortable, confident, and secure during the childbearing process. But, you may be wondering, is an alternative birth as safe as a traditional hospital birth?

IS ALTERNATIVE BIRTH SAFE?

Giving birth in the place where you feel most comfortable and where your emotional as well as physical needs are met can have a profound influence on your labor by reducing fear, tension, pain, the length of labor in some cases, and even complications including fetal distress and cesarean section. In addition, your baby can benefit from a gentle, nontraumatic birth. For healthy mothers, a well-planned alternative birth attended by an experienced, qualified caregiver is in most cases safer than birth within conventional hospital walls.

Because prenatal care, better nutrition, antibiotics, and blood transfusions for maternal hemorrhage have become widely available over the last few decades, the infant mortality rate has dropped. This decrease was paralleled by a higher proportion of mothers who gave birth in hospitals, leading to the assumption that birth in the hospital attended by a physician was safer than home birth for all mothers. However, no study has ever supported this assumption. In fact, as the chapters ahead point out, each of the alternative birth options in this book is usually *safer than conventional hospital birth*. In the alternative-birth setting, the mother is at a reduced risk (and often at no risk) of *iatrogenic* (doctor-caused) medical complications and *nosocomial* (hospital-caused) infection and other problems in childbearing.

The safety of each alternative birth method—home birth, childbearing-center birth, in-hospital alternative birth, midwife-attended birth, and waterbirth—is discussed in detail in the chapters ahead.

WHO CHOOSES ALTERNATIVE BIRTH?

The majority of parents choosing alternative birth have made their choice carefully. They read journal articles, take childbirth classes, and discuss their options with childbirth professionals and other parents. For the most part, they are better-informed than their conventional hospital-birth counterparts.

Every mother—regardless of risk status—can benefit from alternative birth. An essentially healthy mother whose pregnancy has little chance of medical complications is considered *low-risk*. If you are low-risk, you can choose from any of the options in the following chapters. Pregnancy is considered *high-risk* if there are previous medical, current obstetric, or social conditions that are potentially dangerous to the health and/or life of the mother or baby, such as a history of having low-birthweight babies, a maternal illness such as diabetes, or problems that have developed during the pregnancy such as premature labor.

Low and high risk, however, are relative terms. Some health professionals are overly stringent in their definition of low risk. For example, some place all mothers over age thirty-five in the high-risk category even though such women have just as much chance of giving birth normally as anyone else.

Still, not all women are equally safe giving birth at home or in a childbearing center; some are safer in hospitals equipped to handle high risk. If you are considered at high risk of developing complications, your options may be more limited than those of the mother with a completely normal pregnancy. However, you may be able to apply many of the ideas in the chapters ahead to your own situation. For example, in the obstetric department at McMaster's University Medical Center in Hamilton, Ontario, where the latest technological equipment is available for high-risk labors, the mother's other children are welcome. Cribs or cots are brought into the mother's room so the children can stay with her. A cot is also available for the father or birth partner, or he can share the bed with his mate.

Even if you can't find a hospital like this and must give birth in a less-than-ideal setting, you can still work toward making your birth an emotionally rewarding as well as safe event by looking into midwife care, hiring a childbirth assistant, or taking some of the other steps described in the chapters ahead.

The mother is able to give birth in an emotionally positive climate. A safe birth environment is, of course, the prime concern for most mothers. Some parents think this means having medical equipment available. While available medical equipment is certainly a factor in a safe place of birth, safety and an emotionally positive climate also

THE BENEFITS OF ALTERNATIVE BIRTH

Each alternative-birth option discussed in the chapters ahead has its own distinct advantages. Following are some of the benefits common to all.

- an emotionally positive climate for birth
- a more efficient and more comfortable labor
- freedom of mobility throughout labor
- freedom to labor and give birth in the position of the mother's choice
- freedom to breathe and push in harmony with her body's needs
- freedom to eat and drink to satisfy the body's needs
- a reduced need for pain medication
- less chance of unnecessary medical intervention
- a greatly decreased chance of having a cesarean section
- enhanced parent–infant attachment
- the freedom to breastfeed anytime mother and baby want without interruption
- a healthier, happier adjustment to new parenthood
- no unnecessary separation from family members

go hand in hand. The birth environment can influence uterine function, the length of labor, how much discomfort the laboring woman experiences, parent–infant bonding after birth, and even whether or not the mother develops complications.

Many conventional hospital labor and delivery units are not really conducive to normal labor. They are sterile, clinical environments, polluted by the jarring noise of loudspeakers, where the mother is not as comfortable as she would be in a more homelike setting. In addition, the narrow beds common in most hospitals do not permit the mother freedom of movement or allow room for the father to be with his mate, holding, caressing, and supporting her.

The mother is more likely to have an efficient labor. Laboring in a nonclinical environment with an emotionally positive climate often leads to a more efficient labor. This is because the physiology of labor, like that of lovemaking, is influenced by emotions and is frequently affected by disturbances in the environment.

It is well known that labor often slows down and sometimes even stops entirely upon admission to the hospital. Presumably, this is the result of the mother's anxiety in the unfamiliar environment. As Dr. Stanley Sagov, Dr. Richard Feinbloom, and their associates point out in their text *Home Birth: A Practitioner's Guide to Birth Outside the Hospital,* "Some women may react to the stresses of the hospital environment by developing tensions that in turn complicate labor and may therefore require medical interventions that would not have been required in their homes." Of course, a similar argument can be used to justify hospital birth if that is where the mother *feels* most comfortable. In fact, some women's labors don't get going *until* they are in the hospital.

However, in an eye-opening study, Dr. Niles Newton, former professor in the Department of Psychiatry at Northwestern University, found that disturbances in the environment had a significant health impact on laboring mice. A number of mice near delivery were moved every hour or two from a familiar sheltered cage to a glass bowl with cat odor, so that an equal number of mice were always in both bowl and cage. A far greater number of mice delivered in the sheltered cage. In a similar study with laboring mice, researchers found that disturbances contributed to a 65- to 72-percent delay in labor.

The mother has freedom of mobility throughout labor. The United States is one of the only nations in the world where laboring women are expected to stay in bed. This peculiar childbirth custom, common to many hospitals, actually contributes to a longer, more difficult labor. The vertical position increases the speed of labor and reduces discomfort. In alternative-birth settings, laboring women are almost always encouraged to walk around as they feel comfortable.

The mother usually can adopt the position of her choice for labor and birth. Advocates of alternative birth agree that the mother should be free to adopt whatever position she finds most comfortable during labor. This approach has advantages during both first-stage labor, as the cervix dilates, and second-stage labor, during the birth of the baby.

First-stage labor. You will almost invariably adopt the best labor position by following your intuition. Generally speaking, upright positions such as standing, sitting, kneeling on all fours, and walking are best for first-stage labor. Several studies have shown that the vertical position decreases discomfort, increases the speed of labor, and may even decrease the incidence of fetal distress.

Though in some hospitals, the mother is allowed to give birth in a semireclining position, in many hospitals the supine (back-lying) position is preferred, especially when electronic fetal monitoring is engaged. This position, however, can cause maternal hypotension (low blood pressure) as a result of pressure from the heavy uterus on the inferior vena cava and reduce the amount of oxygen reaching the baby, causing fetal distress. The supine position can also lead to less efficient and more painful uterine contractions, as well as a longer labor. In an alternative-birth setting, the supine position is avoided.

Second-stage labor. A large truck tried to pass under a bridge that was too low. The truck got jammed in the center, and its roof wedged against the bottom of the bridge. The truck driver couldn't figure out what to do, nor could the tow-truck driver or the police. While they were standing around talking about removing part of the truck's roof, or even temporarily relocating the girders on the bridge, a little boy came along to watch. The boy said, "Why don't you let the air out of the tires?"

If everyone in this story except the little boy had worked in conventional American maternity units, it is quite likely a similar situation could have happened. Numerous times, I've observed nurses tell a mother to push in a back-lying position when it was obvious she was making no progress. Rarely will conventional hospital practitioners suggest that the mother get up and squat. Yet the birth canal is slightly shortened and the pelvic outlet is expanded by an average of 28 percent in the squatting, as compared to the supine, position. In addition, gravity is on the squatting woman's side. Squatting can shorten an otherwise long bearing-down stage and is especially helpful if the baby is in a posterior position.

Despite this, the most common position for conventional hospital birth remains the supine position. Next to standing on her head, the back-lying position with feet in stirrups is about the worst the mother could assume for giving birth. Stirrups were invented by the ancient Scythians for riding horses, not for having babies. Today, stirrups may be useful for certain gynecological procedures or for the repair of lacerations and use of forceps when truly necessary, but they are best avoided for normal birth. Having your legs in stirrups during second-stage labor makes pushing more difficult and increases the chance of tearing, having an episiotomy, and a forceps delivery.

The supine position is also associated with several risks and disadvantages, including the mother's being forced to push her baby out against gravity, greater difficulty giving birth, increased pain, increased perineal lacerations, and decreased blood flow to the uterus (with its associated potential for fetal oxygen deprivation) resulting from constriction of the mother's blood vessels.

Dr. Roberto Caldeyro-Barcia, past president of the International Federation of Gynecologists and Obstetricians, has stated that, with the exception of being hung by the feet, the supine position (flat on the back with feet in stirrups) is the worst position for labor and birth.

The supine position was first popularized for the convenience of the caregiver, not for the mother's comfort. In contrast to this Western custom, in the majority of nonEuropean-nonAmerican countries, women gave birth in some form of upright position—sitting, squatting, on hands and knees, or standing with support.

The mother is able to breathe and push in harmony with her body's needs. When allowed to breathe with their body's urges, most women do not hold their breath to help push during labor. In many conventional hospitals, however, mothers are enthusiastically coached to take a deep breath, hold it, and push while a nurse or group of nurses does a countdown from five or ten to zero. Such prolonged breath-holding decreases the amount of oxygen that reaches the baby. Fortunately, this practice is falling by the wayside.

Many hospitals and physicians have arbitrary time limits on how long the mother is allowed to push before medical intervention is necessary. At one time, prolonged pushing (greater than two-and-a-half hours) was thought to be related to poorer fetal well-being, increased infection for the mother, and postpartum hemorrhage. Recent research, however, has questioned the need to adhere to such arbitrary time limits for second-stage labor.

The mother is able to drink and eat to satisfy her body's needs. Strange as it may seem, in many conventional hospitals food and a safe place of birth, safety and an emotionally positive climate also was originally instituted when a high percentage of mothers gave birth under general anesthesia, with the accompanying risk of vomiting while unconscious and asphyxiating on the stomach's contents. However, few receive general anesthesia today, and those who do are intubated to prevent such an occurrence. Yet the no-food-no-liquids policy lingers in most hospitals like stale food after a party.

Nurses frequently offer ice chips to laboring women to quench thirst. Ice chips may be welcome, especially if the mother is sweaty, but they aren't much of a substitute for nourishing liquids and a hot meal! Labor is hard work, and you will need and certainly deserve a decent meal. You will especially need nourishment if your labor is long. The traditional hospital IV supplies energy, but it is no sub-stitute for eating and drinking normally. Though it is true that di-gestion may slow during labor, it doesn't stop altogether. (Most women enjoy hot tea with honey or fruit juice. It is best to eat light foods, such as gelatin, hot soup, and toast with jam. Nutrition dur-ing pregnancy and labor is discussed in Chapter 3.) As in most ev-erything else in the alternative-birth setting, the mother's body is her guide about when to eat and drink.

The mother's need of pain medication is usually significantly re-duced. Women who choose alternative-birth methods use dramat-ically less pain-relief medication than mothers who give birth in conventional hospital settings. The use of pain-relief medication is very rare during home birth, and in most childbearing centers pain medication is not even available. However, even in those centers where medication is readily available, women rarely have the need to request it. In one survey of 4,500 women giving birth in a hospital-owned childbearing center, less than 4 percent requested analgesia.

All obstetrical anesthesia and analgesia affect uterine contrac-tions and can impair labor. Epidural anesthesia numbs the body from chest to toes and renders the area temporarily immobile. This form of anesthesia is usually administered when the cervix is di-lated four or five centimeters during first-stage labor. While the mother sits up or lies curled on her side, the anesthetic agent is in-jected into the spinal-canal region. A thin tube is left in the mother's back so more anesthesia can be injected as needed.

Epidural anesthesia is associated with an increased need for Pitocin, a medication used to augment labor contractions (discussed later); an increased need for forceps delivery; more extensive epi-siotomy and lacerations; and a higher rate of cesarean surgery.

According to Dr. John B. Caire of Lake Charles Memorial Hospital in Lake Charles, Louisiana, the use of regional anesthesia (referred to as epidural, spinal, caudal, or saddleblock) reduces labor's effectiveness, causes various degrees of *fetal anoxia* (inadequate oxygen supply), and hinders the bearing-down process.

I recently conducted a workshop for the childbirth professionals in a hospital where 90 *percent* of mothers had epidural anesthesia. Expectant mothers were actually given epidural classes to prepare for its administration. The cesarean rate at that hospital is about 40 percent.

No medication is entirely safe for your baby. In addition, the use of pain medication for the mother frequently breeds more intervention. For example, drugs can slow labor down, causing the caregiver to initiate hormonal augmentation, which in turn may precipitate the need for a cesarean.

The mother avoids unnecessary obstetrical intervention. Obstetrical intervention includes the shaving of the perineal area, administration of an enema, intravenous feeding, electronic fetal monitoring, artificial rupture of the membranes, the use of oxytocic drugs such as Pitocin to augment labor, and the cutting of an episiotomy. Each will be discussed in detail. In many conventional hospitals, all the aforementioned procedures are routine.

In my opinion, the guiding principle in helping women through labor should be "If it works, don't fix it. Otherwise it might really break down." But what actually occurs in many conventional hospitals is a kind of meddlesome obstetrics that often causes more problems—physical and psychological—than it repairs.

According to pediatrician and epidemiologist Marsden G. Wagner of the World Health Organization, "Obstetrical intervention rates in the United States far exceed those of any country in Europe. Indeed, the cesarean section rate in the United States ranges from nearly double to over triple that of the European countries. . . . Countries with some of the lowest perinatal mortality rates in the world have cesarean section rates of less than 10%."

Labor is the only natural process that has been turned into a clinical procedure! Behind the scenes of many conventional hospitals is the view that birth is a medical crisis for which technical help is needed every step of the way. The alternative-birth philosophy is that birth is a natural, normal event that, most of the time, needs no medical intervention. As Dr. G. J. Kloosterman, professor of obstetrics at the University of Amsterdam, puts it: "Childbirth in itself is a natural phenomenon and in the large majority of cases needs no interference whatsoever—only close observation, moral support, and protection against human meddling."

While some procedures may have a place in more complicated labors, they usually have no place in normal childbirth. Routine medical intervention actually can cause the very problems it was designed to prevent. None of the following procedures is routine in an alternative birth.

Shaving the perineal area. Shaving or clipping the hair around the vagina, sometimes called *prepping,* is still routine in a few hospitals, though for the most part, this curious custom is falling by the wayside. In the past, prepping was thought to reduce the chance of infection. However, research reveals that prepping actually may increase the possibility of infection. Further, shaving the pubic hair causes the new mother discomfort while the hair grows back. With a new baby on her hands, the last thing she needs is perineal itch!

Enemas. In some hospitals, the laboring woman is given an enema shortly after admission, though, like prepping, this procedure is becoming less common. The enema's purpose is to clear the bowels prior to birth. However, prelabor diarrhea usually does this effectively. It is common for a little stool to be expressed during birth, which is wiped away and scarcely noticed.

Some mothers find the enema considerably uncomfortable, particularly during late labor. For those who feel they need one, a self-administered enema would be preferable to one administered by a stranger.

Intravenous feeding. Intravenous feeding, or IV, replaces normal fluid and food consumption in a number of hospital labor and delivery units. Those who favor IVs for laboring women claim that they will make it easier to administer medication or an immediate blood transfusion should such be required, which is somewhat like advocating routine intravenous feeding in automobiles, because an accident may occur necessitating blood transfusions. Intravenous feeding has its place in the treatment of the ill. If the mother is unable to take food or liquids by mouth for some reason, the IV may be justified during labor to prevent dehydration or hypoglycemia (low blood sugar). But alternative-birth practitioners agree that IVs have no place in normal labor, during which the mother can eat and drink lightly. The IV makes the mother *feel* like an invalid, impairs her mobility, and by so doing, impairs her labor.

Electronic fetal monitoring (EFM). The electronic fetal monitor (EFM) is a machine that records both fetal heart rate (FHR) and the intensity of uterine contractions on a continuous sheet of graph paper. There are two basic types of monitoring—external and internal.

External monitoring. Two straps, attached to a nearby machine, are placed around the mother's abdomen. On one, an ultrasound transducer picks up the FHR; on the other, a pressure-sensitive device detects the intensity of uterine contractions.

Internal monitoring. A wire is passed through the vagina and cervix and is attached to the baby's scalp to pick up the FHR. A fluid-filled, pressure-sensitive catheter is also inserted into the uterus to determine the intensity of contractions. Often the FHR is monitored internally and contractions are monitored externally. Internal monitoring is more accurate but also more complicated and invasive.

There are two other methods of monitoring the fetal heart: the practitioner *auscultates* (listens to) the baby's heart rate with a special stethoscope called a *fetoscope,* or the heart tones can be heard with a *doppler,* a hand-held ultrasound device that amplifies the fetal heart sounds.

EFM can reveal fetal distress and has a valid place in the obstetrical care of high-risk labors, which is why the monitor was introduced. However, electronic fetal monitors have suddenly appeared in hospitals across the nation and have become routine in normal labor.

According to a report issued by the National Institutes of Health, "Present evidence does not show benefit of electronic fetal monitoring to low-risk patients." In fact, EFM can *disrupt* normal labor. This is, no doubt, the reason the cesarean rate for impaired labor has been shown to be as much as double among electronically monitored mothers.

In an often-quoted study, Dr. Albert Haverkamp and three other physicians divided 483 mothers of similar risk status into two groups. One group had EFM; in the other, a nurse listened to the FHR through a fetoscope. Among the monitored mothers, the cesarean rate was 2½ times higher, with no difference in the baby's well-being. There was also a dramatic increase in postpartum infection among the EFM group.

The results surprised Dr. Haverkamp. He discovered that, contrary to the beliefs of many conscientious obstetricians, EFM is "not associated with an improvement in perinatal outcome." Several other physicians have also clearly demonstrated a correlation between use of EFM and increased cesareans, and a study published in the *New England Journal of Medicine* showed that there was no benefit to the use of EFM during premature labors. In fact, a higher cerebral-palsy rate was observed with the continuously monitored group.

Clearly, there are numerous disadvantages to EFM, which can be summarized as follows.

- The supine position often adopted during EFM can lead to fetal oxygen deprivation.
- EFM inhibits the laboring woman's mobility, which interferes with normal labor and may lead to fetal distress. In addition, the birth partner is inhibited from providing close, caressing labor support when the mother is hooked up to the machine.
- Internal EFM requires rupture of the membranes, which carries its own risk of infection.
- With a belt around her abdomen and a wire running out of her birth canal, the mother's spontaneous reaction to labor is severely inhibited. Drs. Howard L. Minkoff and Richard H. Schwartz have called attention to "the stress a monitored patient may experience because of the use of noisy, incomprehensible machines." Stress is associated with the release of catecholamines (stress hormones such as adrenaline), which may produce vasoconstriction (narrowing of the blood vessels) and reduce heart rate.
- In addition to increased postpartum infection, other risks of EFM include fetal-scalp abscesses and accidents to the baby from internal monitor electrodes.

As if that were not enough, monitors frequently malfunction, giving erroneous information. In fact, I once heard a radio broadcast, rather than the fetal heartbeat, coming from a mother's abdomen!

Despite the studies showing the potential hazards of monitoring, EFM is becoming more, rather than less, popular. One reason is that the machine saves nursing time. Hands-on monitoring with a simple fetoscope or doppler requires care by a skilled nurse. A major advantage of alternative over conventional birth is that women do not need such advanced technical assistance to birth normally.

Artificial rupture of the membranes (ROM). Intentionally rupturing the membranes, also called *amniotomy,* is a common procedure in many hospitals. During this procedure a nurse or the primary caregiver ruptures the membranes (bag of waters) during early or midlabor using either a finger or, more commonly, a long plastic hook shaped somewhat like a crochet needle. This painless procedure is done to speed up labor and/or to attach an electrode for internal EFM.

Numerous researchers have pointed out several disadvantages and risks to both mother and baby associated with artificial ROM. The amniotic fluid provides a sterile environment and cushions the baby during uterine contractions so that pressure is evenly distributed. What can happen when the membrane is ruptured is that the mother experiences stronger, more painful contractions; there can be damage to the soft bones of the baby's skull and also potential oxygen deprivation from compression of the umbilical cord.

ROM also increases the likelihood of having a cesarean section. In most hospitals, once the membranes are ruptured, the clock is set in motion. The mother is generally expected to give birth within twenty-four hours (to reduce the chance of infection) and may be given a labor-inducing drug. In addition, after ROM compression of the umbilical cord and perhaps a fall in uterine-blood flow may contribute to fetal distress, which in turn often results in a cesarean.

Though amniotomy can sometimes shorten labor by about an hour, the results of this procedure are at best inconsistent and unpredictable. Dr. Roberto Caldeyro-Barcia, former president of the International Federation of Gynecologists and Obstetricians and director of the Latin American Center of Perinatology and Human Development for the World Health Organization, points out that "acceleration of labor is not necessarily beneficial for the fetus and newborn and it may be associated with poor outcome for the offspring."

Other, more natural, ways of shortening labor include a vertical rather than horizontal position, the physical and emotional support of a birth partner, and laboring in a peaceful, relaxed setting. Occasionally, however, ROM is beneficial, speeding labor along when other methods won't help. During late labor, some women find rupturing the membranes a relief. But the decision to rupture the membranes should be the mother's.

Use of drugs to augment labor. Labor that stops or slows down is not necessarily abnormal. A few mothers have on-and-off contractions for several days before labor becomes active. Sometimes labor takes a pause, in the manner of a hiker stopping for a rest midway up the mountain. This pause does not mean that labor is petering out or somehow abnormal.

It is often the hospital staff and policies that *cause* labor to slow down. When nurses or physicians stand about waiting for labor to become active, the laboring woman often becomes anxious, wondering if her body is indeed performing correctly. The very pressure to *perform* can impair labor, which is a mind/body process readily influenced by emotional factors.

Furthermore, in many hospitals, labor is expected to progress within a certain time frame. If the laboring woman does not make progress within that time, her labor is augmented with intravenous Pitocin, an artificial form of the pituitary hormone oxytocin, which helps to regulate uterine contractions. Pitocin may be recommended when labor does not progress on its own and there is no other way to precipitate it. However, it does have several disadvantages.

Pitocin-induced contractions are usually more tumultuous and less easy to manage. They seem to rise suddenly to a peak rather than building up gradually, which frequently and understandably creates a need for pain-relief medication. In addition, at most hospitals, mothers who are given Pitocin must also have EFM to record any consequent fetal distress.

Use of oxytocic drugs is frequently the first step in an obstetrical round robin. A woman's labor stops or slows down, often as a result of being admitted to a frightening, impersonal environment. Pitocin is administered to increase contractions, causing more painful contractions. The laboring woman requires pain medication, which further slows her labor. The Pitocin dosage is increased, and the cycle continues until fetal distress is recorded on the monitor and the decision to do an *emergency* cesarean is made. (Of course, the mother will feel grateful that the cesarean was able to *save* her baby, and often doesn't realize that had she given birth in a less clinical, technically oriented setting, the baby might not have been distressed in the first place.)

In addition to sometimes producing fetal distress, Pitocin is associated with an increase in the incidence of jaundice in the newborn and possibly even death.

Several studies have shown that disturbance in the birth place impairs labor and can even affect the health of the offspring. But there are other factors that can prolong labor, including tension between the laboring woman and her birth partner, the presence of someone with whom she feels uncomfortable, physical inhibition, and strong negative feelings about becoming a mother. Labor can often be enhanced by meeting the mother's psychological needs through counseling prior to the birth. If the mother is relaxed, prepared, secure, and in a peaceful environment where she is receiving ample emotional support and knows what to expect, she often is better able to labor more rapidly.

Episiotomy. An episiotomy is often justified if the baby is distressed or in an unusual position, as it facilitates the birth. However, many conventional physicians cut an episiotomy on every mother. They argue that it shortens the birth process and substitutes a neat, easier-to-repair cut for a jagged tear. However, as neat as it may be, the episiotomy is usually far *larger* than most natural tears and more painful during the postpartum period. For that matter, there is often no tearing at all.

Further, the medical literature reveals no support for the routine episiotomies performed by the majority of U.S. obstetricians. In the Netherlands, a country with much less focus on medical intervention during childbirth and a much lower infant-mortality rate, the rate of episiotomy is 6 percent compared to close to 90 percent in the United States.

Most physicians and midwives who practice in alternative-birth settings do episiotomies only rarely, if at all. They are skilled at manipulating the perineal tissue over the baby's head and will use perineal massage and hot compresses to help the woman avoid tearing. Even more important, they have learned to trust the mother's body to give birth without unnecessary surgery.

The mother has a dramatically reduced chance of a cesarean section. Because of certain conditions a cesarean section is recommended to preserve the health or life of a baby or mother. These conditions include:

- placental abruption, in which all or part of the placenta separates from the uterine wall. If the abruption is complete, a cesarean is performed to prevent maternal hemorrhage and fetal death.
- placenta previa, in which the placenta covers all or part of the cervix at the time of birth. A cesarean is performed to prevent severe maternal blood loss and fetal death.

- umbilical-cord prolapse, in which the umbilical cord precedes the baby in the birth canal. In this condition, the baby's oxygen supply is cut off and a cesarean is usually necessary to prevent brain damage or death from asphyxia.
- malpresentation, in which the baby is in other than the vertex, or head-down, position. In the breech position—buttocks or feet first in the birth canal—the baby often can be delivered vaginally, though this is associated with a higher percentage of complications. The baby in the transverse lie—shoulders first in the birth canal—cannot be delivered vaginally.
- an active case of genital herpes. While passing through the canal, the baby can become infected, leading to damage or death.
- diabetes mellitus. There is a higher risk of fetal death during the last few weeks of pregnancy with diabetic mothers. Accordingly, a preterm cesarean often is done if the condition is severe.
- other maternal illnesses. A few illnesses contribute to serious complications for either mother or baby including pre-eclampsia/eclampsia (a pregnancy disease characterized by hypertension, swelling, and protein in the urine), chronic hypertension (high blood pressure), and certain cardiac and kidney diseases.

If you have one of these conditions at the time of giving birth, you may need to have cesarean surgery. However, the overwhelming majority of cesareans performed in the United States are unnecessary.

Since the 1960s, the U.S. cesarean rate has more than quadrupled, and is one of the world's highest at 25 percent, meaning one in every four mothers gives birth via major abdominal surgery. (By comparison, in the Netherlands, the rate is about 7 percent.) In some hospitals, the cesarean rate is as high as 30 or even 40 percent.

I believe that it is best to avoid surgical birth whenever possible. Cesarean surgery is associated with a constellation of physical and emotional problems which I call *surgical birth trauma.*

Surgical birth trauma, affecting the entire family, consists of:

- the unique physical problems of the cesarean mother, including a slightly higher risk of maternal mortality; a higher

percentage of postpartum illness, particularly infection; increased risk of hemorrhage; injury to adjacent organs during the operation; aspiration pneumonia; postoperative gas pains; and a far longer, more uncomfortable postpartum recovery period.
- maternal–infant separation and its consequences (discussed in the next section).
- the emotional consequences of cesarean birth, which affects both parents. Some parents feel grief, disappointment, frustration, guilt, or a sense of inadequacy and failure.
- the unique physical problems of the cesarean-born baby, which include an increased risk of respiratory distress syndrome, jaundice, and other problems.

The mother who gives birth at home, in a childbearing center or attended by a midwife has a far lower chance of unnecessary surgery than the mother who plans a conventional hospital birth. A recent study of childbearing centers nationwide showed the cesarean rate to be 4 percent—less than one-sixth our national average.

Mothers who have had cesareans often wonder whether they can give birth to their next child vaginally. Not long ago, vaginal birth after a previous cesarean (VBAC) was actually considered "alternative birth." VBAC was so outside the mainstream that many mothers had difficulty finding a caregiver who would assist them with VBAC; some still do. Today, however, we know that VBACs are safer than repeat cesareans for most women. The medical profession is slowly coming to accept VBAC as the standard of care for previous cesarean mothers.

For more information on preventing an unnecessary cesarean and preparing for a vaginal birth after a previous cesarean, please see the suggested reading at the end of this book.

Parents and baby remain together and are likely to experience enhanced parent–infant attachment. Routine separation of mother and baby during the hours that follow birth has to be one of the most unfortunate customs of modern times. In many hospitals, the newborns are taken to a central nursery, where they usually shriek at the top of their lungs, and the mothers are taken to recovery rooms where—if she is not in a drugged stupor—she almost invariably worries about her child.

Animal breeders wouldn't think of handling a birth in such a manner. They don't separate animal mothers and babies, because they know that to do so would have long-term detrimental effects on both. We are just now beginning to learn what farmers have known for centuries.

Pioneer researchers Drs. Klaus and Kennel, who published the results of their ground-breaking research on the subject of maternal–infant attachment, have called attention to the fact that the immediate postpartum period is an emotionally very sensitive time in the development of *bonding,* that is, the development of parent–infant attachment. A study conducted at Duke University in North Carolina showed that the breastfeeding rate increased over 50 percent when mothers had no option but to room in with their infants. Infants who had immediate postnatal contact with their mothers tended to have fewer infections for the first year, to gain more weight, and to be breastfed longer.

In one study comparing couples planning home birth, natural hospital birth, and anesthetized hospital delivery, psychotherapist Gayle Peterson and her associates showed that parent–infant attachment seemed to be enhanced by home birth. Research has also revealed that mothers who have prolonged contact with their infants shortly after birth demonstrate greater affection and attachment for their babies later on. Similarly, there is a proven greater percentage of neglect, abuse, and failure to thrive among infants who are separated from their parents shortly after birth.

Hospital practices, such as routine maternal–infant separation and separation of mother from her family, often seriously interfere with the parent–infant attachment process. Fortunately, maternal–infant separation (except in medical emergencies requiring immediate pediatric attention) is becoming a thing of the past as more and more health professionals realize how detrimental it is to the entire family. Further, though this sensitive postbirth period should not be interrupted unless necessary, love can't be reduced to a series of biological patterns. If you aren't able to spend the first postnatal hour with your child for any reason, you will still develop parent–infant attachment.

Parents and infant almost always remain together without interruption in an alternative-birth setting. All medical procedures (which include weighing, measuring, use of eye drops to prevent gonococcal infection, and possibly administration of vitamin K, as well as taking a blood sample for routine tests) are usually delayed for at least an hour while parents and newborn get to know one another. Both mother and father can hold the baby. I usually recommend that the father remove his shirt and hold his newborn against his bare chest for a few minutes, covering the baby's back with a blanket for warmth. This skin-to-skin contact enriches the father's birth experience.

Though bright light may sometimes be necessary to examine the baby's color, in the alternative-birth setting practitioners recognize that the room should be dimly lit after a child is born. This is in striking contrast to the often brightly lit hospital delivery room. Leaving the womb is probably a little like stepping out of a low-lit room into a sunny outdoors: the blinding light hurts, and the baby's eyes screw shut in reflex.

If the lighting is low, the baby will open his or her eyes, look around, and usually lock eyes with the mother and father. That first moment of eye contact is magical. Waves of nameless feeling swept up and down my spine when I first locked eyes with my newborn son.

The mother is able to breastfeed spontaneously and without inhibition. Immediate postbirth breastfeeding is practically the rule in the alternative-birth setting, as it is common knowledge that breastmilk provides far better nutrition than formula for premature as well as full-term babies. In addition to meeting all the infant's nutritional needs, it protects the baby against a host of allergies and diseases. The premilk substance called *colostrum* helps the baby to clear excess mucus from the mouth and throat while supplying antibodies to a host of diseases, particularly of the intestinal tract. Another advantage of breastfeeding is that when the baby sucks the breast, the pituitary gland releases the hormone oxytocin, which causes the uterus to contract, thereby facilitating the delivery of the placenta and helping to prevent postpartum hemorrhage. And finally, breastfeeding has been shown to have long-term psychological benefits for the child.

Yet many hospital routines and practices are inimical to breastfeeding. For example, babies are often placed in a central nursery, separated from the mother. There the baby is frequently given water or formula, interfering with the breastfeeding pattern. Also, many maternity nurses use alcohol wash, which can cause the mother's nipples to dry, crack, and bleed. When the mothers do breastfeed, it can be painful.

The parents are likely to have a healthier, happier adjustment to new parenthood. Many, if not the majority of, American mothers suffer some form of "baby blues"—that constellation of tears, irritability, and depression that begins about the third to fifth day after birth and continues for a period of anywhere from a couple of days to several weeks. I have heard childbirth educators tell parents that this is a normal, almost inevitable part of childbearing.

While changing emotions is natural after having a baby, baby blues doesn't have to be inevitable. Conventional hospital practices contribute to the condition. According to Helen Varney of the Maternal-Newborn Program at Yale University's School of Nursing, "Postpartum blues are largely a psychological phenomenon of the woman who is separated from her family and her baby."

The blues are less common after an alternative birth. British pediatrician Aidan Macfarlane says that depression occurs in about 60 percent of mothers who give birth in hospitals but in only 16 percent of mothers who give birth at home.

There are a couple of reasons for this. First, at home, mother and baby are not separated during the sensitive period immediately following birth. Second, in the home—as in other alternative-birth settings—a woman makes the most natural transition possible to becoming a mother. She is already in her own home, and there is no separation from her family.

The mother can remain with her family. Avoiding prolonged separation of the new mother and her family can mean a healthier adjustment for everyone. Though some mothers want their birth to be a private event shared just by their mate, others view birth as an experience to be shared by the entire family and, often, close friends.

For many laboring women, family and friends at birth lessens fear. Continous emotional support of loved ones is almost invariably associated with a more comfortable labor. In addition, being surrounded by familiar faces assists many women to better surrender to labor.

The mother should have the final choice about with whom she wants to share her birth. However, many hospitals restrict the number of people she can have with her during labor. Some don't even allow the father to attend unless he has taken special childbirth classes. Ironically, most hospitals that deny the laboring woman the guests of her choice have no trouble accommodating medical and nursing students.

I have visited hospitals that advertise themselves as offering "family-centered maternity care" yet don't even allow children to be present during the first hours after the baby is born, let alone during labor. Children are part of the family, and many parents feel it is important that their other children participate in their brother or sister's arrival in the world. Sibling involvement at birth or during the immediate postpartum period may enhance siblings' acceptance of the newcomer and decrease trauma.

Whether or not the family opts to have the children at the actual birth, they should certainly be included immediately afterwards. They should be allowed to hold and touch the baby—not simply to view him or her through the glass window of a nursery.

In alternative birth settings, there are no restrictions on the participation of family. In fact, this is one of the primary reasons many families choose alternative birth—in a hospital, a childbearing center, or at home—over conventional labor and delivery.

A FINAL WORD

When a child is born, a woman and a man cross the one-way bridge to become mother and father. A baby makes the greatest of all passage rites from life inside the womb to life in the world. An alternative birth can make that life-altering transition smoother for the entire family. It can make the mother's postpartum recovery easier and happier, and it can enhance the love bond both parents have with their new child. For these reasons, alternative birth can have a long-term positive effect on the entire family.

Certified nurse-midwife Elizabeth Hosford, past Coordinator of the Maternity Center Association in New York City, and her husband decided on a home birth for her first baby over two decades ago. She writes: "It never occurred to either of us that it was anyone's right but ours to make that decision. . . . It came as a bit of a shock to me in my egocentric pregnancy ecstasy to learn that we were subjects of sharp censure by medical colleagues who assumed it was *their prerogative* to determine what should happen to us and our baby—and where!

"I felt then as I do now. It is my inalienable right to determine where, with whom, and how I shall bear my children so long as I do it within the realm of safety. Freedom of choice with all its implications cannot help but bring a new level of quality to family-centered care. And a new level of optimism across the land."

As more parents learn about the benefits of alternative birth, I believe that the options discussed in this book will become more common than conventional hospital birth. When this occurs, alternative birth will no longer be considered "alternative"; it will be the norm.

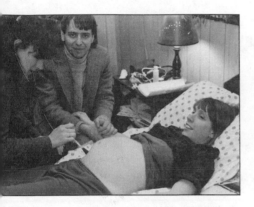

CHAPTER 2

A Safer, More Positive Labor: A New Model of Childbirth

EVERY YEAR THOUSANDS OF NEW mothers leave hospitals frustrated, angry, and sad about their birth experience. Many feel cheated of the joy that a safe, positive birth can offer. As was noted in Chapter One, one out of every four mothers in the United States has a cesarean section, even though the overwhelming majority of these operations are unnecessary. Many of these mothers are disappointed and are depressed for days, weeks, or even months after the cesarean is performed. An estimated 60 to 80 percent of American mothers experience some form of "baby blues," a constellation of negativity, tears, frustration, and depression. Yet this phenomenon is largely the result of unnatural birth customs and therefore often avoidable.

The disappointment most mothers experience with contemporary childbirth can be dramatically reduced by adopting a model of labor and childbirth that encompasses the mother's mind and emotions as well as her body. In most alternative-birth options, the mother's emotional and psychological as well as physical needs are addressed. Her family's needs are addressed as well. As the noted psychologist Dr. David Chamberlain has so beautifully pointed out in his ground-breaking book *Babies Remember Birth,* the baby is a conscious and sensitive participant in the childbearing process. In an alternative birth, the baby's emotional as well as physical needs are considered. The father too is usually viewed as an integral part of the childbearing process.

Alternative-birth options are therefore more satisyfing for the entire family. In addition, with few exceptions, for the healthy mother a well-planned alternative birth is safer.

This chapter will examine the experience of labor and childbirth as a mind/body process. Adopting a model of childbirth embracing both body and mind is the single most important step you can take toward creating a safer, more fulfilling birth experience.

A MIND/BODY PROCESS

Labor is a mind/body process. The experience of labor consists of a series of both physiological and psychological changes that occur as labor progresses.

There is really nothing "new" about this perception of labor: midwives have realized the mind influences labor and that labor influences the mind for centuries. Nevertheless, many childbirth educators teach expectant parents only about the physical process of labor—the changes that take place in the cervix and the way in which the baby is born. This is a tale half-told. We can no more understand the experience of labor by hearing about cervical dilation than we can get an idea of what lovemaking is like by reading a technical article on pressure and release.

Mind and body are inextricably linked during labor. Giving birth involves the whole being—body, mind, and emotions. As labor progresses, the laboring woman experiences profound psychological changes. Her consciousness is altered and passionate emotions are released.

We know that the mind and emotions influence a wide range of physiological processes from digestion to blood pressure. Lovemaking is the only other physical function as readily influenced by thoughts and emotions as labor. Your emotions not only affect whether or not you have a positive birth experience; they also affect the relative amount of pain you experience in childbearing, the length of your labor, and, to a degree, your baby's well-being.

Whatever influences the laboring mind also influences the laboring body. This includes the birthing environment, the caregiver, others attending the birth, the support the mother receives from her birth partner, and the mother's own feelings about birth. Understanding this is the foundation for preparing for a positive birth experience.

In this section I will first present the physical process of labor, then discuss how the mind and emotions are affected as labor progresses.

THE PHYSICAL PROCESS

During pregnancy, your body prepares for the amazing process that will bring your child into your waiting arms. The uterus, shaped like an inverted pear, expands to contain a full five hundred times its prepregnant capacity. Its sturdy muscular walls thicken to keep your baby snug and secure in its temporary home and to push the baby to the world outside when it is time to give birth. The cervix—the neck of the uterus, which protrudes into the vagina—softens from a cartilaginous consistency similar to the tip of the nose to something as soft as an earlobe, *effaces* (thins), and sometimes begins to *dilate* as much as one to four centimeters. By the end of the third trimester, the cervix is *ripe,* that is, partially effaced, dilated, and ready to open a gateway for the baby during labor. The vagina, whose velvety walls have shaded from a delicate pink to a rich violet during the prenatal months as a result of an increased blood supply, also prepares to stretch. The connective tissue softens and the delicate folds of mucous membrane that make up the vaginal walls prepare to unfold.

During labor, the powerful uterus rhythmically tightens and relaxes. These rhythmical tightenings, or labor *contractions,* occur intermittently until the baby and placenta (afterbirth) are born. Labor contractions are often compared to ocean waves. Each builds, reaches a crest, and ebbs. At labor's beginning the waves are usually gentle, like ripples; toward labor's end, they become more powerful, like the waves of a stormy sea.

Every labor is unique. One mother may labor for two or three days with contractions occurring in an on-and-off pattern, while another may have intense contractions and labor from start to finish in four hours. However, all labors have three stages.

First-stage contractions efface and dilate the cervix until it is wide enough for the baby to be born. Cervical dilation (often spelled *dilatation*) is measured in centimeters (abbreviated *cm.*). The cervix is said to be fully dilated at approximately ten centimeters (about four inches). As dilation takes place, contractions also push the baby downward so that the cervix begins to stretch over the baby's head like the neck of a tight sweater.

The first stage of labor can be divided into three phases:

Early-labor (to 4 cm. dilation) contractions are usually mild, last from thirty to forty-five seconds each, and occur at decreasing intervals from about every twenty to about every five minutes.

Active-labor (from 4 to 7 cm.) contractions may last from forty-five to seventy-five seconds each and occur at decreasing intervals from about every seven to about every two minutes (the average being five- to three-minute intervals).

Transition (from 7 to 10 cm.), also called *late active-labor*, contractions may last from sixty to 120 seconds and occur at variable intervals ranging from about every three to two minutes.

The total length of first-stage labor may be any time from two to three hours to thirty-six hours or longer. The average length is about twelve hours. Labor is usually, but not always, shorter for second-time mothers.

Second-stage labor is the birth of the baby. This begins when the cervix is fully dilated. The mother usually feels an urge to bear down and push her baby out. The second stage may last anywhere from a few minutes to several hours, the average length being from one to two hours.

Third-stage labor is the delivery of the placenta. Its average duration is from ten to fifteen minutes.

The Experience of Pain in Labor

The degree of pain in labor varies from one woman to another. A few women experience almost no pain, but most find labor hard work, and usually painful. As one mother put it: "It was difficult but never more than I could bear."

Labor is not continuously painful. The mother experiences the most discomfort during contractions, and the pain of contractions varies throughout labor. Generally speaking, contractions that occur toward the end of the first stage are considerably more painful than those at the beginning.

The second stage usually feels quite different from the first. It can vary widely, from being "intensely difficult" to being "exquisitely pleasurable." For some mothers, the actual birth process is as painful, if not more so, than the first stage. For most, however, the second stage is less painful. In one mother's words: "It was incredibly exciting! The pain of contractions left when the cervix was fully dilated."

Third-stage contractions are often barely noticeable in the excitement of holding the new baby.

The pain of labor is different from other kinds of pain you may have experienced. Many have described it as "positive pain," a contradictory-sounding expression that refers to two things. First, labor contractions are purposeful; the pain is "healthy" pain. Each contraction brings the mother a little closer to her goal of seeing her baby. At the same time, the strong, powerful contractions of the late first stage massage the baby and prepare her for her first breath. Second, though it is painful at times, most mothers find labor a rewarding, fulfilling experience—something no one would say about a toothache!

As you'll see in the chapters ahead, giving birth in an alternative-birth setting where your emotional as well as physical needs are fulfilled can dramatically reduce the pain of labor and heighten your joy in birth. In addition, there are two effective means of reducing the fear and pain of labor without drugs. One is being well-supported by a nurturing mate or birth partner, as discussed in the pages ahead. The well-prepared father or birth partner is, as one nurse put it, "worth his weight in Demerol." The second is using guided imagery, a technique that will be explored in Chapter Three.

Labor encompasses a wide variety of feelings, from agony to ecstasy. If it were solely an unpleasant experience, we would not hear so many new mothers, radiant with joy, exclaim: "I want to do it again!"

THE LABORING MIND RESPONSE

While the cervix is dilating during first-stage labor, the laboring woman experiences a series of dramatic psychological, emotional, and behavioral changes. Taken together these make up what I call the *laboring mind response.*

I developed the concept of the laboring mind response for two reasons. First, I wanted to give expectant parents and childbirth professionals a description of the *experience* of labor, rather than the mere physical process. My goal was to convey—in simple, down-

THE STAGES OF LABOR

Stage/ phase of labor	Cervical changes	Length of contractions	Interval between contractions	Duration of stage/phase
First Stage				2 to 36 hours
Early labor Latent Phase	Cervix effaces and dilates to 3 to 5 cm.	Increasing: 30 to 45 seconds	Decreasing: 20 to 5 minutes	6 to 8 hours
Active Phase	Cervix dilates from 3 to 5 to 7 to 8 cm.	Increasing: 45 to 75 seconds	Decreasing: 7 to 2 minutes (average 5 to 3 minutes)	2 to 3 hours
Transition Phase	Cervix dilates from 7 to 8 to 10 cm.	Increasing: 60 to 120 seconds	Variable: 3 to 2 minutes	½ hour to 2 hours
Second Stage	Birth of baby	60 seconds	Variable: 5 to 2 minutes	A few minutes to 2 or more hours
Third Stage	Delivery of placenta	Variable	Variable	10 to 20 minutes

For first-time mothers, the average duration of first-stage labor is 12 ½ hours. For those who have given birth before, the average is about 6 hours. The average duration of second-stage labor is 1 ½ hours for first-time mothers and ½ hour for those who have given birth before.

The information in this summary is based *only on averages*. The length of individual contractions and the duration of each phase may vary widely and yet still be perfectly normal.

(This chart is adapted from *The Birth Partner's Handbook* by Carl Jones, Meadowbrook, 1989, page 21.)

to-earth language—the laboring woman's altered state of mind, as well as the psychological and behavioral changes that occur as labor progresses. The idea for the laboring mind response came about while I was giving workshops to childbirth professionals and heard many describe how difficult it was to teach parents about these aspects of labor.

Second, I wanted to explain why guided imagery was an effective means of reducing the fear and pain of labor. Many childbirth professionals who attended my workshops knew that guided imagery worked from their own personal experience using the method with laboring women, but few understood why it was so effective.

The laboring mind response consists of seven characteristics that most women experience to a greater or lesser degree. Being familiar with these characteristics will give you insight into the labor experience and will enable you to make birth plans (such as choosing a birthing environment) that are most conducive to a safe, rewarding labor.

I strongly urge the father or other birth partner, as well as the mother, to learn about the laboring mind response. This will help him better understand his mate's experience so he can provide effective labor support, reducing the mother's fear and pain. For this reason, I have shown how each of the following seven steps applies to the birth partner.

1. *The right brain takes precedence.* As labor progresses, the focus of the laboring woman's energy seems to shift from the left hemisphere of the brain to the right. The left hemisphere is associated with logic, reasoning, and analytical thinking. The right hemisphere (sometimes called the *heart brain*), on the other hand, is associated with creative and artistic thinking, intuition, love-making—and labor. As the right hemisphere comes to dominate the scene, the mother becomes more intuitive, emotional, and instinctive.

The birth partner who is aware of the laboring woman's right-hemisphere orientation will be better equipped to provide the emotional support and encouragement that she needs. It is important for him to understand, for example, that giving his mate emotional support is often more effective than giving her a series of instructions.

2. *The laboring woman is in an altered state of mind.* The mother may greet labor's onset with any of a wide variety of reactions—she may be anxious, elated, relieved, or excited. Regardless of these responses, she may be able to function normally and

continue with her everyday life. Once labor is underway and contractions continue to dilate the cervix, however, she experiences a profound psychological transformation. Her consciousness will be altered, as if the contractions that are opening the cervix are also opening a primal part of her mind.

Along with her greater right-hemisphere orientation, the mother becomes less rational, more instinctive, and more intuitive. She seems to enter her own world. As one father put it: "It was as if she were in a different world traveling in a new dimension as she lay in my arms." Expressing a similar idea, Dr. Richard B. Stewart of the Birthing Center at Douglas General Hospital in Douglasville, Georgia, says, "If you provide the proper environment, a laboring woman will go into her own psyche and shut out the external world."

As a result of their temporarily altered consciousness, many mothers forget to do things they have planned. For example, a mother may forget something she has learned in childbirth class about coping with contractions, or a mother who plans to view the birth in a mirror may forget all about this when the time comes. Her birth partner can help by reminding her of what she has planned.

The laboring mother's concentration will narrow as she becomes more introspective. Her contractions and those persons in her immediate environment become her world. The birth partner's presence, love, and support will assist the mother to yield to the psychological changes labor triggers and thereby experience a less painful and more efficient labor.

One new mother told me, "I never understood what you meant by the laboring mother's altered state of mind until I was in labor. Then it all made sense to me!" I have found this to be true of many women. The mother—to say nothing of the father—often has no clear picture of labor until she is actually experiencing it.

3. *The laboring woman experiences altered perceptions of space and time.* As labor moves along, the mother's perceptions of space and time seem to become progressively distorted. It is not uncommon for the laboring woman to think her contractions are lasting much longer than they actually are.

The laboring woman becomes wholly caught up with the forces that are bringing her child into the world. Odd as it may sound, some women even lose sight of the fact that they are going to have a baby! It is as if, in her profoundly altered mind, the mother temporarily forgets the purpose of what she is experiencing.

The birth partner can best support the mother through one contraction at a time. He can also occasionally remind her she will soon see her baby.

4. *The laboring woman experiences heightened emotional sensitivity.* As labor progresses, the laboring woman becomes highly sensitive, vulnerable, and dependent on her birth partner and those around her. Almost all mothers experience this heightened sensitivity toward the end of first-stage labor.

At the same time, the mother's emotions influence her labor. It is extremely important that parents and professionals be aware of this characteristic of the laboring mind response. A disturbance in the environment actually can cause labor to slow down. It is well known, for instance, that contractions often slow down and sometimes peter out altogether when the mother enters the hospital.

The birth partner who is aware of the profound impact emotions have on labor will be able to significantly reduce the mother's fear and pain by being an emotionally nurturing and supportive presence.

5. *The laboring woman usually has lowered inhibitions.* Social inhibitions tend to be dramatically reduced during the course of labor. For instance, the laboring woman may remove all of her clothing as labor nears its end. She may groan, moan, and sigh. She often becomes unconcerned with who sees her unclothed body or hears the sensual sounds she is making. This behavior is especially common at home or in a childbearing center, because the alternative setting is usually most conducive to a normal and spontaneous reaction to labor.

The birth partner should realize that this is normal behavior, to be encouraged. It is a sign that the laboring mind response has been elicited.

6. *The laboring woman exhibits distinctly sexual behavior.* Lovemaking and labor are obviously poles apart; sex is associated with pleasure and labor with pain. However, since both labor and lovemaking take place within the sexual organs, labor is a sexual process. This does not mean labor is a sexual *experience,* or necessarily pleasurable.

There are striking similarities between the two processes. The following list is based on my own observations of laboring women combined with those previously noted by other childbirth professionals.

- During both labor and lovemaking, the uterus rhythmically contracts, though the contractions are far more intense during labor.
- During both processes, the vagina lubricates and opens.
- Both are associated with the right hemisphere of the brain.
- During both labor and lovemaking, a woman becomes intensely emotional and vulnerable.
- Emotions influence both processes. Disturbances, emotional conflicts, and inhibitions can impair both.
- Social inhibitions decrease during both labor and lovemaking.
- A woman has a similar expression near sexual climax and toward the end of labor.
- During both processes, women often make similar sounds— moaning, sighing, or groaning.
- Both processes are often followed by a state of well-being.
- Both are *primal* processes that are most satisyfing when a woman surrenders body, mind, and emotions to the experience.

Surrendering to labor, letting go, yielding to the experience is the key to a smoother, less painful, and more rewarding birth experience. In other words, the same conditions that are conducive to satisfying lovemaking are conducive to a safe, positive birth experience. These include peace, privacy, comfort, subdued lighting, freedom from disturbances, the ability to surrender to the process, and a setting where the woman is free to react spontaneously.

Understanding this characteristic of the laboring mind response will enable the birth partner to better relate to the mother's "sexual" behavior. For example, he should be aware that groaning, sighing, and moaning do not necessarily indicate pain. The sensual sounds the mother makes are part of the natural voice of the laboring woman; they well up from the soul. Accepting this behavior as normal will assist the mother to more easily surrender to labor.

I often point out that the vagina lubricates and opens during labor as it does during lovemaking. Labor also triggers a psychological as well as physiological opening. "You want to open for your baby like you open for your lover," I often suggest to women in my workshops.

Laboring women appear to sense the need to open on a deep, intuitive level. The very word *open* has almost magical power during active labor. The birth partner can use a soft, soothing voice to tell the mother to think of herself opening and to imagine her cervix dilating as well. This often causes a difficult labor to progress more rapidly. Another good way to do this is to use the "Opening Flower" imagery exercises mentioned in Chapter Three.

7. *There is increased openness to suggestion.* During active labor, the laboring woman becomes more easily influenced by suggestion than perhaps at any other time in her waking life. For example, a caregiver, impatient for labor to be underway, might enter the room and say, "Your labor is progressing slowly." Though such a simple suggestion would probably have little or no effect during ordinary life, once the laboring mind response has been elicited, the suggestion may actually cause the mother's contractions to slow down.

Toward the end of labor, suggestions seem to have a magnified impact on the woman. The good news is that this applies to positive as well as negative suggestions. Comments such as "You are really doing fine!" or "You can do it!" can help the mother better cope with labor. Likewise, the positive suggestions of guided imagery can have a powerful effect on helping the mother through labor. The birth partner should be as positive as possible in his words and actions.

Being familiar with the laboring mind response will enable you and your mate to better cope with labor and make birth plans more conducive to a rewarding childbearing experience. For example, if you recognize that labor triggers profound emotional and psychological changes, you will be likely to choose a physician or midwife with whom you feel psychologically compatible. With the assumption that medical competence is the only important factor, many pregnant women don't put this kind of thought into their choice of caregiver, and this can lead to a disappointing birth experience. You have a far greater chance of a positive birth if you select a caregiver who understands your emotional as well as physical needs, or who at least respects your individual goals regarding childbearing.

You will also see the need to select an emotionally positive birthing environment where you feel free to experience a spontaneous reaction to the laboring mind response. Some parents feel that creating such an environment—which is an integral component of alternative birth—is not as important as the health of mother and baby. However, maternal–infant health and the fulfillment of the mother's emotional needs are inextricably linked.

THE LABORING MIND RESPONSE

As labor progresses, most women experience the following seven characteristics to a greater or lesser degree.

- right-brain dominance
- an altered state of consciousness
- altered perceptions of space and time
- heightened emotional sensitivity
- decreased inhibitions
- distinctly sexual behavior
- greater openness to suggestion

The father who is acquainted with the laboring mind response will be better able to provide effective labor support. For example, he will be able to see why caressing the laboring woman and giving her verbal encouragement in a soft, soothing voice is often more effective than "coaching" her with regulated breathing. Above all, he will recognize that the most powerful support he can give is his love.

A POSITIVE VIEW OF BIRTH

A positive view of birth is the cornerstone for preparing for a safe, rewarding alternative-childbirth experience. The mother who believes that her body was designed to give birth normally is more likely to have a smooth labor than the woman who believes that giving birth is a potential disaster. In my opinion, there are four beliefs essential to a positive image of birth. These are:

1. Childbirth is a normal, healthy event, not an illness. No one, of course, actually thinks that childbirth is an illness. However, many parents and professionals *act* as if it were.

The fact that birth is unconsciously linked with images of disease is one of the major reasons conventional medical practitioners often frown upon alternative birth. In this society, the laboring mother is often cast in an invalid role, helpless and in need of hospitalization. This peculiar custom has affected the birth experiences of millions of mothers. Educating parents and professionals about alternative-birth options begins with believing that birth is a healthy, normal process.

2. *Birth is a natural process, not a medical event.* Though it sounds absurd to remind anyone that birth is natural, this seemingly obvious fact needs to be reinforced—particularly in the United States, with its nearly 25 percent cesarean rate and high rate of obstetric intervention. In modern society, birth is largely viewed within a medical frame of reference. For many parents and professionals childbirth conjures up images of women with IVs, electronic fetal monitors, and assorted other medical equipment. While medical intervention is sometimes necessary, today, with our emphasis on medical technology, we often lose sight of the birth process itself.

Appreciating that birth is a *natural* process doesn't necessarily mean the mother is committed to laboring and giving birth with no medication. Rather, it implies that she accepts that birth, like conception, is a physiologically natural process.

3. *Childbirth is a social event.* By this expression, I am referring to the fact that birth is the beginning of a family, and this is a significant social transformation in the lives of most couples. In addition to the mother's giving birth, labor is an awesome passage rite for the entire family. The baby makes the dramatic passage from life inside the uterus to life in the world. A man and woman cross the one-way bridge to become a mother and a father, and another child becomes a brother or sister.

I often encourage parents to think of their birth as they would their wedding. You should make it just as special, just as beautiful.

4. *You, the parents, are the center of the childbearing drama.* The mother *gives* birth. Although her caregiver, nurses, and whoever is attending the birth may be able to help in a variety of ways, it is the mother whose strength and power bring the child into the world. Similarly, it is the father's strength and power that will reduce the mother's fear and pain and help her experience a safe, fulfilling birth.

As it is the parents who are the center of the childbearing drama, they, not the medical staff around them, should be in charge. This is one of the many points that distinguishes alternative-birth options from conventional hospital delivery. And when this is so, the mother is often less tense and more able to react spontaneously to labor. Labor goes more smoothly because her mind and body are working in harmony.

HOW THE CHILDBIRTH EDUCATOR CAN HELP

You have already seen how understanding the laboring mind response can better enable parents to prepare for a safe, rewarding birth and reduce the fear and pain of labor. Adopting this model of childbirth can also help childbirth educators and health-care providers better meet expectant and laboring women's needs.

The childbirth educator has a vital role in preparing women and their birth partners for a safe, positive birth. A good instructor can give the parents a clear idea of what to expect in labor, acquaint them with their choices in childbirth, and teach effective ways to cope with the labor. However, many parents leave childbirth classes without having learned about *any* of these topics.

Adopting a mind/body model of childbirth could revolutionize childbirth education. Teaching the laboring mind response in addition to the physical process of labor would enable instructors to better prepare parents for birth in four ways.

1. *The childbirth educator would give parents a much clearer picture of labor.* "I was totally unprepared for labor!" exclaimed one new mother who had taken eight weeks of childbirth classes. "The instructor taught tons of breathing exercises but didn't give me the slightest idea of what labor would be like."

I hear this kind of comment all the time. A childbirth educator who covers the physical process but fails to talk about the *experience* of labor is like an aerobic-exercise instructor giving a lecture about the anatomy and physiology of respiration without doing any exercises.

In my opinion, covering the emotional changes labor triggers is even more important than teaching about the mother's bodily changes. After all, the parents don't see the cervix dilate, but they *do* see and experience the laboring mother's altered state of mind and altered behavior.

2. *The childbirth educator would be more likely to inform parents about their options in childbirth.* This would enable the parents to select the birth method with which they feel most comfortable. Acquainting parents with their birth options is an integral part of good childbirth education. Women will feel safest and most secure in a variety of different settings. For this reason, I believe every childbirth educator has an obligation to present home, childbearing-center, and hospital birth as equal choices. However, many educators discuss only hospital birth.

3. The childbirth educator would better prepare the father for his support-giving role. A number of childbirth educators refer to the father as the "labor coach." In all my workshops, I urge childbirth professionals not to use this misleading term. Birth is not an athletic event but a natural, normal process.

Some women prefer their birth partner to give them instructions. However, even this preference does not mean the father should be cast in the "coach" role. Such a role encourages fathers to dominate and control the mother's reactions to labor—the very approach which is best avoided. It can also distance the father from the childbearing miracle. Being a coach is much like being behind a camera, instead of being part of the event.

The childbirth educator who understands the laboring mind response will encourage the father to be nurturing, to maintain physical closeness with his mate, and to be emotionally supportive, in addition to teaching him a wide variety of comfort measures such as massage for back pain.

4. The childbirth educator can give the parents more effective ways to cope with labor. There are two effective ways to reduce the tension, fear, and pain that, I believe, should be added to the curriculum of all childbirth classes. These are helping the mother surrender to labor and teaching her and her mate to use guided imagery.

Surrendering, yielding to the mind/body changes of the laboring mind response, is the key to letting labor work in the most efficient possible way. This does not mean that the mother cannot distract herself from pain with methods like concentrating on a focal point, regulating breathing, or chanting, but implies that she should accept as a normal process the psychological and emotional changes labor precipitates.

A Better Health-Care Professional

Contemporary obstetrical care is based on a thorough knowledge of the anatomy and physiology of childbirth. Without question, this is a necessary component of medical care through pregnancy, labor, and the postpartum period. However, since the mind influences the body during labor, medical care for the laboring mother's body is only half the picture. As British psychotherapist Bianca Gordon points out: "Whether or not a mother's experience of childbirth is a happy one depends not only on the physical care she receives but also on the care for her emotional needs, and on recognition of her as a unique individual."

In conventional medical practice, childbirth is approached as if it were a medical event, a procedure such as an appendectomy. Many, if not most, physicians know nothing about the emotional changes the laboring woman experiences. They are unaware that the mind influences labor. In fact, astounding as it may seem, many obstetricians *have never attended a single labor.* During medical training, the medical student or resident occasionally checks on the laboring woman and attends medical procedures but does not actually sit with the woman throughout her labor.

In the chapters ahead, you will read about professionals who have helped many mothers enjoy rewarding, fulfilling birth experiences in alternative-birth settings while maintaining safety records far superior to most national averages. These are the exceptional caregivers. Some women travel for miles, even across the country, to give birth under their chosen professionals' care.

What makes these caregivers different from the conventional physician is that they acknowledge that labor is a mind/body process. If this acknowledgment were more universal, it would enable all childbirth professionals to provide care conducive to the laboring mother's needs, thereby increasing the likelihood of a safer birth for mother and baby. The physician who realizes that the laboring woman experiences heightened emotional sensitivity will try to create an emotionally positive environment rather than simply provide a setting with all the latest medical equipment available. Similarly, the caregiver who understands that labor is a sexual process will provide a setting and style of health care conducive to letting go and surrendering to the life-creating miracle of birth.

LOOKING AHEAD

To reduce the experience of labor to a description of how the cervix dilates and how the baby descends in the birth canal is like trying to capture love in a test tube. There is more to giving birth than the observable realities of hard science. Labor affects the mother's whole being—her mind and emotions—as well as her body. Realizing this is, in my opinion, the key to understanding what makes alternative birth more rewarding than conventional hospital delivery.

Conventional obstetrics, by focusing on the physical experience alone, is robbing the experience of birth of its beauty and individuality. Alternative birth, which encompasses the emotional as well as the physical dimensions of childbearing, has reconnected us with the heart and soul of giving birth and the spontaneity and sexuality of the laboring woman.

I have tried to explain some of the psychological aspects of labor through the discussion of the laboring mind response. There is yet another facet of labor that cannot be reduced to a formula, seen on a monitor, or measured in a laboratory, and that is its essential mystery. We can approximate in words the physiological, psychological, and emotional changes the laboring woman experiences, but can we explain what takes place when what was a tiny seed makes the awesome passage rite to becoming "my son" or "my daughter"? That is something that must be experienced to be felt. And even then, it remains a mystery—perhaps the greatest mystery of all.

In my opinion, adopting a new model of childbirth based on understanding the psychological as well as physical process of labor is the most significant step we can take toward a safer, saner obstetrics. Reeducating modern medical professionals will no doubt take much time. But, for now, there is something you can do to help.

After you've read this chapter, have your caregiver read it.

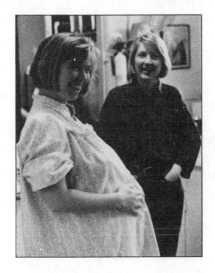

Preparing For Your Alternative Birth

WHETHER IT TAKES PLACE AT home, in the childbearing center, or in a hospital, a safe, positive birth depends largely on healthy prenatal habits and good preparation. Though you may not be able to eliminate all the discomforts of pregnancy and labor, you will increase your chance of enjoying a healthier, happier pregnancy and birth if you observe the following steps.

- Get regular prenatal care throughout pregnancy.
- Eat nutritiously.
- Exercise regularly.
- Plan your birth carefully.

PRENATAL CARE

The person who will be attending your birth—whether it be physician or midwife—will generally provide prenatal care. However, if you haven't yet chosen your caregiver, go to a physician, midwife, or clinic for prenatal care and then, if you have found someone you

45

prefer, switch caregivers when you make a final choice. If someone other than the person who will be attending the birth is providing your prenatal care, get a copy of your medical records for the caregiver who will be your birth attendant.

Your first prenatal visit should be a get-acquainted session. Discuss your birth plans (if you have already made plans) and your feelings about the type of care you would like in labor. Become acquainted with the caregiver's philosophy of childbirth. Some caregivers do not automatically provide routine get-acquainted sessions, so it's best to state your preferences over the phone when you make your initial appointment.

After the initial consultation, your first prenatal appointment will probably include a complete medical history and physical exam; a pelvic exam to confirm pregnancy, to assess the size and shape of the pelvis, to take a Pap smear, and to test for gonorrhea (some caregivers, however, wait until the final trimester to do a pelvic exam); a breast examination; weight measurement (to determine weight gain throughout pregnancy); and a blood test, checking blood type and RH factor, for anemia, syphilis, and other infections and for German measles immunity, and confirming pregnancy. Subsequent prenatal visits will usually include a blood-pressure check, a weight check, a urine analysis, a check of the growth of your uterus, and a fetal-heartbeat check.

Begin prenatal care by the third month of pregnancy to be sure your pregnancy is progressing normally or to spot possible complications.

Attend prenatal appointments with your mate if possible. During one of my workshops in which I had been encouraging childbirth professionals to invite the father to prenatal appointments, a midwife said, "I don't just invite fathers to come, I demand it! 'You showed up at conception,' I tell them. 'I expect you to show up here!' "

The father needn't attend every exam if he doesn't want to, but he should certainly be present at a few. "We thought of our pregnancy as a joint venture," recalls Janet, a new mother. "Kevin attended all prenatals with me; it seemed right for him to share as much as possible."

Though it will probably mean taking time off work (unless the caregiver has evening hours), the benefits of father-attended prenatals will more than outweigh the inconvenience. There are several advantages:

- The father is able to evaluate the caregiver and have a part in deciding whether or not to hire this person.
- He learns more about the pregnancy and becomes more involved.
- His presence often helps the mother feel more secure, comfortable, and at ease.
- He can listen to the baby's heartbeat.
- He can ask questions and air his own concerns.

Attending prenatal appointments together will assist both parents in planning their birth. As Kathy Kangas, mother of three and director of Childbirth Education Services in Worcester County, Massachusetts, recalls: "It was great support to have Tyler at appointments with me. We felt we were creating our birth together."

EATING NUTRITIOUSLY

When you're pregnant, your nutritional requirements increase over those of the nonpregnant woman in order to meet the needs of your own tissue growth, your increased metabolism, and the needs of your developing baby. Eating well is directly related to your baby's well-being and essential to the needs of your changing body. A host of complications can be prevented by observing good nutrition during pregnancy.

Your caloric needs will probably increase by about 300 calories daily. Every calorie should count. Avoid empty-calorie junk foods as well as highly processed foods with low nutritional content. Snacks between meals should be healthy and nutritious, such as raw fruits and vegetables, nuts, raisins, a little cheese, and granola bars. Cut down on foods like cake, pie, and potato chips.

Your protein needs will also increase. Increased protein intake helps your baby gain weight, and low birth weight has been linked to a variety of complications. Therefore, you should increase your daily servings of complete protein sources such as meats, fish, and eggs. Vegetarian protein sources include lentils, beans, nut butters, nuts, grains, tofu, and sunflower seeds. If you are deriving your protein from vegetarian sources, be sure you are eating complete proteins with all the amino acids. Most vegetarian sources have to be complemented with others; good combinations include rice (preferably brown rice) and lentils; rice and wheat; rice and beans; beans and wheat; soybeans, rice, and wheat; and soybeans, sesame and wheat. It's a good idea to consult a vegetarian cookbook if you plan a vegetarian pregnancy and to discuss your diet with your caregiver.

Your calcium needs will also increase to meet the needs of fetal development and growth of your baby's bones and teeth. You should drink as much as one quart of milk daily or consume its equivalent in the form of cheese, cottage cheese, or yogurt. Other good sources of calcium include tofu, oatmeal, green leafy vegetables, and eggs.

As a result of hormonal change, increased uterine size, and decreased gastrointestinal movement, prenatal constipation is common. To avoid this, include plenty of roughage and fiber in your diet: whole-grain breads and cereals, seeds and nuts, bran (you can add this highly nutritious item to other foods or eat bran muffins if you aren't fond of plain bran), dried or fresh fruit, and raw vegetables with the skins and peels on (if appropriate). In addition, drink six to eight glasses of water or other fluids daily.

With a 40-percent or more increase in prenatal blood volume and the baby's storage of iron, you will also require much more iron than you did before pregnancy. Iron-deficiency anemia, with symptoms including paleness and feeling tired and weak, may result from inadequate iron in your prenatal diet. Natural iron sources include red meats, liver, egg yolks, blackstrap molasses, and green leafy vegetables. Cooking foods in a cast-iron pan will also increase iron contents, and iron supplements are usually recommended. Some expectant mothers find that these contribute to constipation. However, taking supplements at mealtime with citrus fruit or a glass of orange juice will help to alleviate the problem. Folacin or folic acid is also often prescribed during pregnancy to prevent anemia. Natural sources of folic acid include liver, brewer's yeast, and green leafy vegetables.

It is best to eliminate alcohol consumption, as alcohol has been associated with abnormalities in fetal growth. The precise limit of safe alcohol intake during pregnancy is unknown and for this reason, many childbirth professionals suggest eliminating all alcoholic beverages during the prenatal months. Others suggest drinking in moderation, such as a glass of wine once a week. Check with your caregiver for his or her recommendation.

Everyone these days realizes that smoking is a health hazard, but it poses special problems in pregnancy. It has been linked with underweight babies as well as an increase in infant mortality. In fact, pregnancy is an ideal time for *both* parents to quit smoking, since even inhaling your partner's smoke is unhealthy.

Many physicians fail to stress the importance of a healthy diet to their clients. Oddly, not many years ago obstetricians started telling pregnant women to restrict weight gain, some even insisting that they gain no more than twenty pounds. However, consider this: a baby weighs an average of seven to eight pounds; a placenta, one to two pounds; the amniotic fluid, two pounds; the increase in breast weight, two pounds; the increased blood supply, three pounds; retained fluids, another three pounds; fat stores, five to nine pounds; and increased uterine musculature, about two more pounds. Thus the total extra weight is twenty-five to twenty-nine pounds. When I told my seven-year-old son that some doctors suggest that mothers gain less weight than the combined total of the above, he wrinkled his brow and said, "Don't they teach them math in school?"

There is no ideal weight gain applicable for all expectant mothers. Today most childbirth professionals agree that a twenty-four- to forty-pound gain is normal. Some mothers gain more, some less. My wife, Jan, for example, gained only twelve pounds during her first two pregnancies. The pregnancies were perfectly normal, and both babies were in the seven-pound range and quite healthy. But this is the exception rather than the rule.

Let your body be your guide. Eat balanced, healthy, fully nutritious meals. Ask your caregiver for nutritional information if you are unsure whether or not your diet is adequate.

GETTING REGULAR EXERCISE

Childbirth is a demanding physical process requiring all your energy. A mother in good physical condition is more likely to have a shorter, more comfortable labor than one in poor shape. Regular exercise will help reduce common pregnancy discomforts such as backache, heartburn, constipation, leg cramps, and fatigue, and keeping fit during pregnancy will enable you to recover your nonpregnant shape more rapidly after the baby is born.

Aerobic exercises that focus on the respiratory and circulatory systems, such as hiking, bicycling, and swimming are ideal. Many health clubs and gyms have special exercise classes for pregnant women.

Throughout the prenatal months you are able to do almost everything you could before pregnancy, though your sense of balance may not be as stable. However, you should avoid beginning unfamiliar strenuous activities and, of course, you should avoid potentially dangerous activities such as rock-climbing. Consult your caregiver for exercise advice tailored to your needs and to determine when in your pregnancy it's best to moderate the amount of exercise.

During our first three pregnancies, regular mountain hiking kept both my wife and me in shape and doubtlessly contributed to Jan's comfortable pregnancy and her smooth labor.

PLANNING YOUR BIRTH

Planning your birth carefully will help you reduce the fear and pain of labor; have a safer, more fulfilling birth; and enjoy healthier, less stressful days after the baby is born. Ideally, you should start to plan your birth during the early months of your pregnancy. However, many, if not most, expectant parents don't learn about all available childbirth options until late in pregnancy (if at all)—a good reason to keep an open mind until you are sure your birth plans are the best you can make.

Once you have chosen the alternative-birth option that best suits your needs (which I hope this book will help you to do!), the essential concerns in your birth plan are:

- your choice of caregiver
- your choice of health-care options
- the role the father will assume
- your choice of baby's caregiver
- who will attend the birth (siblings, relatives, friends, childbirth assistant)
- your choice of a childbirth class
- your preparation for labor
- getting some help at home after birth

Each of these concerns will be examined carefully.

Choosing a Caregiver

Whether physician or midwife, a good caregiver is a guardian of a natural process, present to assist when needed and to intervene only if necessary. Keep this idea in mind when selecting the person who will help you at your birth.

The most important thing to look for in your choice of caregiver is, of course, medical competence. Ask relevant questions to be sure the person who gives prenatal care and who attends your birth is able to handle an emergency should one arise. For instance, if you are planning a home birth, you might want to find out how many home births the caregiver has attended. Can the caregiver handle complications? What equipment does he or she bring? Can he or she do suturing should you need a laceration repaired?

Most midwives will work with an assistant. There is much to do during labor, and an assistant's hands are usually needed. Be sure to meet the assistant as well as the primary caregiver.

Though of primary concern, medical competence is not the only important issue. Select a caregiver with whom you are reasonably compatible. After all, you are inviting this person to share one of the most intimate events of your life. You want to share it with someone you like and whose philosophy of childbirth is close to your own.

Of course, in many areas it may be difficult to find a choice of caregivers. But if you do have several options, consider the following points.

- Choose someone who supports your individual goals.
- Meet and discuss your birth plans with the caregiver before making a final choice. Your first appointment should be a getting-acquainted session, not an exam. This gives you a chance to determine whether or not you are compatible.
- Be sure your caregiver has adequate backup by a physician (if the caregiver is a midwife) and a nearby hospital (if birth is to take place at home or in a childbearing center).
- Feel free to change caregivers at any time during pregnancy if you are uncomfortable with your present physician or midwife. It is always better to change—even the day before labor begins—than to continue to visit a caregiver who doesn't

wholly support your plans. You needn't have a completely rational reason for changing. You may simply *feel* uncomfortable with your present caregiver.

Remember, *both* parents should feel reasonably compatible with the caregiver. If the father is uncomfortable with the midwife or physician, this may diminish his own experience of the birth. In addition, if he's uneasy, this will be communicated to his mate and may make her uneasy as well. For example, Brenda and Larry, a couple in central Vermont, changed caregivers because their midwife had a strong prejudice against male birth attendants. "She said she believed the father's place was at his mate's side during labor and had no problem with fathers at birth," Larry recalls. "But her anti-male birth-attendant bias seemed to color her entire practice. I didn't feel right paying someone a fee who had this kind of problem with men in her profession."

MIDWIFE OR PHYSICIAN?

Many expectant parents feel most comfortable with a midwife at their birth, whereas others prefer an obstetrician or a family practitioner. Actually, you can have both. The midwife/physician team is an ideal birth-attendant partnership. The midwife provides care for healthy pregnant and laboring women, while the physician is present in case complications arise.

In some areas, the certified nurse-midwife (CNM) attends home births. The CNM is trained in a hospital setting and has much experience. However, this background gives some CNMs an overly clinical view of birth.

The well-trained "lay" midwife can also be a highly competent birth attendant. Many midwives who are trained through a combination of apprenticeship and midwifery school view birth as a natural process rather than a medical procedure. However, if you choose a lay midwife, it is imperative to be sure she is highly qualified.

MALE OR FEMALE?

After a workshop where I had been describing how labor affects the mind as well as the body, a midwife turned in an evaluation with the following comment: "I can't believe it! I never realized a man could actually understand labor!"

Many people—childbirth professionals as well as laypersons—believe that women make better nurses, midwives, child-birth assistants, and primary caregivers than men. This is similar to the old-fashioned prejudice that kept women from medical school. The qualities of the caregiver are what count, not the gender.

I too once thought that a woman—by virtue of her having given birth—would have greater insight into the labor experience and be more sensitive to another woman's needs than a man. However, experiences at scores of births has taught me this isn't so. The fact is that men can be just as sensitive and nurturing as women at birth. Likewise, there are insensitive caregivers among both genders. So have an open mind when choosing your caregiver.

Selecting Health-care Options

When you plan your birth, you will probably find it helpful to draw up a written health-care checklist, or birth plan, for you and your caregiver to follow. It will make you more aware of your options and help you clarify your preferences regarding important details of obstetric and pediatric care during labor, birth, and the early postpartum period, and it will serve as a communication tool conveying your plans and preferences to anyone giving prenatal care, attending your birth, or providing baby care.

A checklist will also help you make contingency plans for the unexpected, such as a transfer from home to hospital, a cesarean section, or unforeseen emergencies. If a transfer from home to hospital must be made during labor or an unexpected cesarean birth becomes necessary, both parents are bound to be overwhelmed. Making the contingency plans *now* can help you avoid much anxiety and the need to make decisions at the last minute.

Discuss the items on the list with your caregiver and ask to have a written list included in your chart. You may want to ask your caregiver to sign the checklist, giving his or her approval of your preferences. Make copies of the checklist for your caregiver, the person providing backup care, and your baby's caregiver. This will heighten your chance of having the birth experience you planned for.

Remember that all expectant parents deserve to be able to create the birth they desire and have *all* their preferences honored whether giving birth at home, at a childbearing center, or in a hospital. Unfortunately, however, many parents are not able to have everything they want. Whether or not you will depends largely on the hospitals and health-care practitioners in the area where you live. Unless you are willing to go to great lengths to fulfill your goals (such as by temporarily relocating), you may have to be flexible about some details.

Following are some suggested items to include on your checklist. These details reflect the personal preferences of many parents who have planned an alternative birth. However, you should create your own list based on your personal preferences.

FOR LABOR AND BIRTH:

- The father (or birth partner) and mother are free to remain together without separation for any reason.
- The parents' birth companions (siblings, family, friends) or childbirth assistant are free to remain with them through labor and/or birth as the parents choose.
- If planning a home birth, the home-birth midwife is free to remain with the parents throughout hospital admission, labor, and birth, should there be a transfer from home to hospital.
- Electronic fetal monitoring is to be done only if there are signs of fetal distress.
- Use of an IV (for intravenous feeding) is to be reserved only for emergencies.
- Only a minimum of internal exams are to be performed.
- No pain-relief medication is to be administered unless the mother requests it.
- No episiotomy is to be cut unless there is a clear case of fetal distress, shoulder dystocia, or some other medical emergency requiring a surgical incision.
- The mother is free to shower and bathe as she wishes (whether or not her membranes have ruptured).
- The mother is free to drink fluids and eat lightly as she wishes.
- The mother remains free to walk around during labor.
- The mother is free to labor and give birth in the position of her choice.
- Labor and birth are to take place in the same room.
- The father is able to assist in the delivery or "catch" the baby.

- The mother is able to reach down and complete the delivery as soon as the baby's head and shoulders are born.
- The father is able to cut the umbilical cord.
- The mother is able to deliver the placenta spontaneously, without uterine stimulants.

For the Immediate Postpartum Period:

- The parents and baby are to remain together without interruption for at least one hour unless there is a medical emergency requiring immediate pediatric attention.
- The parents are free to dim the lights to enhance early parent–infant eye contact.
- The mother is able to breastfeed immediately after giving birth.
- The use of eye drops to prevent infection and the administration of the vitamin K shot are to be delayed for at least one hour following birth.
- Routine baby-care procedures such as weighing, measuring, and footprinting are to be delayed at least one hour following birth (and are to be done only if the parents choose).
- All baby care—including the newborn exam—is to take place in the parents' presence.
- No bottles of formula or water are to be given to the baby at any time during the hospital stay (if you give birth in a hospital or are transferred to one).
- Siblings and other family members are allowed to greet the baby face-to-face within the first hours after birth.
- The mother and baby are allowed twenty-four-hour rooming-in, if birth is in a hospital.
- The father is free to remain with the mother and baby twenty-four hours a day.
- The mother and baby are discharged within twelve to twenty-four hours after birth unless there are medical complications.

For Cesarean Birth:

- The father is free to remain with the mother throughout surgery and preferably throughout preoperative procedures.
- The mother is given options regarding type of anesthesia.

- The mother is given the option of whether or not to take any preoperative or postoperative medications.
- The father may hold the baby close to the mother immediately after birth unless there are life-threatening complications requiring immediate pediatric attention.
- The mother has one or both hands free (rather than strapped to the operating table) to caress her child.
- The father is free to accompany the baby to the intensive-care nursery if there is a medical emergency requiring immediate pediatric attention.
- The father is free to remain with the mother in the recovery room.
- The mother and baby are allowed twenty-four-hour rooming-in.
- The father may remain with the mother throughout her postpartum hospital stay twenty-four hours a day.
- No bottles of formula or water are to be given to the baby at any time during the hospital stay. The baby is breastfed exclusively.
- The mother is discharged within forty-eight hours if she wishes to go home and her condition warrants it.

Planning for the Father's Role

The father can participate in childbearing in a wide variety of ways, from just observing the birth to "catching" the baby as it is born.

The father's *primary* role during labor is to experience the birth of his own child. At the same time, he can tremendously reduce his mate's fear and pain and make her feel more confident, secure, and comfortable. There is no right or wrong way for the father to be involved: he should take on whatever role is comfortable for him and his mate.

Some fathers just want to be present while another family member, a friend, or a childbirth assistant gives active labor support. "I asked other people for support with the breathing and relaxing," recalls Jean, who has had one hospital and three home births. "Tony didn't feel comfortable doing all that. He just wanted to be there. And that was really the best thing for me, just to have him with me."

Other fathers want to give the primary labor support. If the father chooses to do this, he can either be the sole support person or be the main support person while another family member, friend, or professional gives backup support. Regardless of the role he elects to take on, every father should be thoroughly familiar with effective ways of reducing his mate's fear and pain.

Some fathers want to "catch" their own child, and this can be a wonderful experience. The caregiver usually assists with the delivery of the baby's head, that part of birth most in need of expert assistance; then the father completes the delivery. As the baby is born, the mother can reach down, take the child under the arms, and bring the baby to her breast.

Whatever role the father assumes, I do suggest that he cut the umbilical cord. The bluish-white cord is curly, like the receiver wire of a telephone. One end is attached to the baby and the other to the placenta inside the mother, but cutting it does not hurt either mother or baby. The cord will continue pulsing for a while after birth as blood passes from the placenta to the baby. Clamping and cutting should be delayed until the pulsing ceases unless there is a medical reason for doing so immediately. The birth attendant will first prepare the cord by clamping it on either side of the area where it is to be cut, and the cord is then cut with a sterile pair of scissors. I think of cord cutting as a dramatic ritual concluding the passage rite of birth. It is a little like putting the ring on the bride's finger.

THE WELL-INFORMED BIRTH PARTNER
I agree. Nothing can better relieve the mother's fear and pain in childbirth than a nurturing, well-informed birth partner. There are four essentials that will enable the father to give effective labor support and enhance his own experience of the birth.

- *Learning about the laboring mind response* (discussed in Chapter Two). Though the father should learn something about the anatomy and physiology of labor, it is more important for him to have some insight into his mate's changing behavior and altered state of mind.
- *Being nurturing.* The most valuable aid to the laboring mother is her birth partner's ability to give emotional and physical support through such activities as hugging her, caressing her, and massaging her if she requests it.
- *Learning about relaxation and guided imagery.* This is discussed in detail later in this chapter.

- *Learning other ways of making the mother comfortable,* such
  as giving her a back rub, wiping her brow with compresses,
  helping her change position, and responding to any of her
  requests. (I have written two books just for birth partners.
  See the suggested reading list at the end of this book.)

Choosing Your Baby's Caregiver

The caregiver who attends your birth will do a newborn exam. But
you will also need a caregiver for your baby during the weeks and
months following the birth. Now is the best time to choose that
caregiver. You may choose a pediatrician or a family practitioner,
or you may prefer a well-baby clinic for general health care and a
pediatrician for backup should consultation with a specialist be
necessary.

When selecting your baby's caregiver, choose someone who
supports your chosen method of giving birth. Choose a caregiver
who fully supports 100-percent breastfeeding, if this is how you
plan to feed your baby. You might ask what percentage of his or her
clients breastfeed. Look for someone who answers your questions
to your satisfaction and who shares your philosophy regarding cir-
cumcision, immunizations, and whatever other aspects of baby
care are important to you. (For more information on these subjects,
see the suggested reading list at the end of this book.)

Other points to consider are whether or not the caregiver
charges for phone consultations, whether he or she accepts insurance reimbursements (and, if so, whether or not the caregiver charges
for filling out insurance forms), and, of course, how well you get
along. Like selecting the caregiver who will attend your birth, you
and your mate should choose your baby's health-care provider together.

Who Will Attend the Birth?

Some expectant parents elect to give birth without anyone, even a
caregiver, present. Others prefer to have just their caregiver present. Still others want family, friends, and additional support persons to share the event.

If you choose to share your birth experience with others, be
sure everyone who attends is fully supportive of your chosen method
of childbirth. Being surrounded by supportive loved ones can em-
power a mother and make her feel secure. The stress and tension of

having people present who think your birth method—for example, home birth—is tantamount to giving birth in the jungle, on the other hand, can cause you to have a longer, more difficult labor.

FAMILY AND FRIENDS AT BIRTH

An increasing number of expectant parents invite family and sometimes friends to share their birth. The presence of family and/or friends helps some mothers relax, feel more comfortable, and feel greater support during labor. It enables the mother to experience the highs and lows of labor with familiar faces.

"I had everyone under the sun at my birth because it was something I wanted to share with a lot of people," recalls Kathy. "My mother-in-law came to take care of my other child, Mandy. I wanted to give her the gift of watching her grandchild being born. I wanted my sister and sisters-in-law there so they could see exactly what childbirth was like. I also invited my brother-in-law; a friend who was training to be a midwife; and the two midwives who were my primary birth attendants and an extra one who was just there to give support and observe."

Most childbearing centers place no restrictions on whom the mother invites to share her birth. And, of course, she can invite whomever she wants into her home. Hospitals, however, vary in their policies about the presence of others during labor. Some permit only one person to remain with the mother during labor; a few place no restrictions on the mother's guests. If you are planning a birth with others present, select a birth place that honors the mother's right to choose the guests of her choice.

Plan and discuss what role each person attending your birth will assume, from observing to helping out. Guests can help out in a wide variety of ways, from taking photographs, to replenishing warm compresses, to giving emotional support, to preparing a meal to celebrate the event. Make sure your guests are aware that they will be expected to help out.

CHILDREN AT BIRTH

"My daughter, four years old, sat next to me and held my hand during my labor," recalls one new mother. "At the last minute, she asked if she could let go and watch the baby being born and help Daddy and the midwife catch the baby."

Though always a miracle, when seen through a child's eyes, birth is especially magical. From tiny beginnings an unknown being grows in Mom's stomach. During labor the baby leaves its snug and secure home to make a far more fabulous journey than could be made on the wings of a stork. One physician who attends both home and hospital births said that births with children present were the most unforgettable of all he attended. Many childbirth professionals who have witnessed sibling-attended births agree.

When a child becomes a sibling, life changes dramatically and irreversibly. The child must make tremendous adjustments. He or she will no longer have the exclusive attention of Mom and Dad but will learn to share their love. Involving children through pregnancy, birth, and the immediate postpartum period can ease this transition.

During birth, children can help out in a variety of ways, depending on their age. A child can fan the mother, hold her hand, give her ice chips, serve her food and liquids, and assist the father by replenishing hot or cold compresses and doing other odd jobs as the need arises.

Your child should be able to come and go so that he or she does not have to be cooped up in one room for an extended period. A birthing center or hospital with a separate play area for children is ideal, but a hospital lobby, cafeteria, and the street outside can provide needed distractions. Another adult or an older child should be present to care for children under four. Such children may want or need to leave the birthing place from time to time, especially if your labor is long.

Many parents are surprised to discover how children take the childbearing drama in stride. When well-prepared, most children take labor and birth for granted, and little is as wondrous as the face of a brother or sister during the unfolding miracle. Birth through a child's eyes is like Christmas morning. The room seems to pulse with energy, and there is no question a miracle has occurred.

Preparing Children for Birth

My son Carl, age nine, recalls how he felt at the birth of his brother Jonathan.

When my brother, Paul, and I found out we were going to have a new baby in the family, we all started preparing. We read books about how babies grow inside their mothers and how babies are born. Mom and Dad showed us pictures of babies being born so we would know what to expect.

We went shopping for baby clothes and other things. Sometimes that was fun. And sometimes it was real boring.

Paul and I went to the midwife's appointments with Mom and Dad. We heard the baby's heart beat!

The night before the baby was born, I visited my grandma's while my brother, Paul, stayed home. Before I went to bed, I reminded Grandma to wake me up if my Mom went into labor. When she woke me up in the middle of the night, I didn't know where I was at first.

We rushed to our apartment. Grandma drove fast. She went through a red light!

When I got there, the baby was already born! I was sad because I wanted to see the birth. But I was also real excited. I woke up Paul. We both saw Daddy cut the umbilical cord.

And now we are getting ready to have another baby!

When we were preparing for Jonathan's birth four years ago, our three-year-old son, Paul, said, "I want to be a mommy too!" I'll always remember how he cried when we told him boys couldn't be mommies.

We involved both our sons early in our preparation for our third child. We began by asking them how they felt about having a new brother or sister. Once the baby was conceived, they were actively included through the pregnancy and postpartum weeks. Taking the following steps will help prepare your child for birth and the transition to becoming a brother or sister.

Choose a caregiver and, if you are planning an out-of-home birth, childbearing center or hospital supportive of children at birth. Before finalizing your birth plans, be sure your caregiver and, if you are planning a childbearing-center or hospital birth, the staff at your birth place welcome children at birth. Remember, even some hospitals that call themselves "family-centered" do not allow children at birth.

Phone the caregiver or childbearing center and ask how many parents elect to have their children present during labor. You might also want to ask what suggestions they have for preparing a child

for birth. Should the reaction be less than positive, consider another caregiver and birth place if you live in an area where choices
are available.

Some parents choose their birth place for the sake of being
able to have their children present. Helen's story is an example.

The mother of four boys, Helen was pregnant with her fifth
child (whom she hoped would be a girl!). The first four births had
taken place in a local hospital. But this time, Helen wanted a family
birth with her four sons present. Since no hospital in her area allowed children to attend births, she planned a home birth. When it
was time to push her baby out into the world, Helen lay back on her
bed propped up on pillows like a queen. The father sat next to her
and rubbed her back. The four boys at the end of the bed were
breathless, anticipating the birth of their sister.

As the baby's head started to show, the boys were wide-eyed
with awe. The rest of the body slipped out. There was a moment of
silence. Then four grins broke across the boys' faces and their soft
chuckling filled the air.

The mother reached down to take her child. "Oh my God!"
she hollered as she took her fifth son lovingly to breast.

Educate your children about birth. "How is the baby going to pop
out?" our three-year-old son asked. He could understand how the
child grew in the mother's uterus, but how it would get out was another matter. Paul was not alone. Even though they are acquainted
with the anatomy of birth, most mothers and fathers wonder the
same thing!

Tell your child what to expect during labor and birth, being
sure to include the delivery of the placenta. Let your child know
that there will be a considerable amount of blood so the blood will
not be a surprise.

Be sure to mention how some mothers moan, sigh, and even
scream at times.

Some childbirth educators hold sibling-preparation classes.
Some classes are designed to prepare a child for becoming a brother
or sister but not necessarily for attending the birth; others prepare
the child to participate in the birth. You may want to consider
bringing your child to one of your own childbirth classes. This can
be helpful especially if a birth film is shown. If you would like to
view such a film, call local childbirth educators (see Resources) and
ask if they have one that you can arrange to see.

After the twentieth week of pregnancy, with a hand on the mother's abdomen, your child can feel the baby move. For siblings, this can be a turning point marking the time when the pregnancy stops being a big belly and becomes a little brother or sister.

Give the child a realistic idea of how newborns look and behave. Explain that they don't look much like the babies in baby-food ads for the first weeks of life. Furthermore, children should know that newborns are not very exciting playmates. Many children are disappointed to find that the newborn is interested only in eating and sleeping. However, you can involve your children in the infant's life. Depending on your child's age, you can acquaint him or her with ways to help out, from changing diapers to sharing a bath with the newborn.

Include your children at prenatals. As pregnancy unfolds, your child should meet your caregiver. At prenatal appointments, the sibling-to-be can listen to the fetal heartbeat through a *fetoscope* (a special stethoscope designed for hearing fetal heart tones). He or she can also ask questions. Several midwives and physicians have birth picture books the child can look at to learn about the birth process while waiting for the exam. If you are planning to give birth in a childbearing center or hospital, take your child to visit the birth place. Seeing where Mom and Dad will be acquaints the child with what to expect.

Shopping for the layette. Shopping for the baby clothes, toys, and furniture can also help a child of any age adjust to the fact that there will be a new family member. Psychiatrist Martin Greenberg, whose pioneer research in the area of paternal–infant bonding is well known, told me that while shopping for the layette with his wife he was utterly surprised to see how tiny newborn clothing was. It was a striking confrontation with how vulnerable and dependent his new child would be. If a physician who is intimately acquainted with newborns finds the size of infant clothing a surprise, imagine how a brother- or sister-to-be feels!

Shopping for the layette is a good opportunity to explain that the newcomer will be wholly dependent on its mother for a while and will therefore need the lion's share of attention. This is an important issue to confront before your baby is born, and conveying it to your other children will make your life more comfortable and more serene afterwards.

The Childbirth Assistant

Many expectant parents hire a childbirth assistant (also known as a CA) to give labor support in place of or in addition to the father. These childbirth professionals are called a variety of peculiar names, including "monatrice," "coach," and "doula"—none of which actually describe what the childbirth assistant does.

Childbirth assistants are usually nurses, midwives-in-training, childbirth educators, or laypersons. Most have special training and experience in giving labor support as well as assistance during the early postpartum period. One organization, the National Association of Childbirth Assistants (NACA), conducts workshops to train both health professionals and laypersons to become childbirth assistants.

In many birth settings, the childbirth assistant is the *only* person who remains with the parents throughout labor and the early postpartum period. Most physicians are present only during the final part of labor, to assist during the birth. As a general rule, midwives remain with the laboring mother for a longer time, though usually not throughout her entire labor. In most hospitals, nurses come and go as the shifts change. The childbirth assistant, on the other hand, is a familiar face from the beginning to the end of the mother's labor.

The childbirth assistant can offer perspective, reassurance, encouragement, and suggestions. She is an invaluable assistant to home VBAC (vaginal birth after cesarean) mothers, single mothers, and others who simply want the presence of another knowledgeable person besides their caregiver.

Some CAs can check blood pressure and fetal heart tones and do vaginal exams to assess cervical dilatation. Some give support only during labor; others give postpartum assistance and breastfeeding advice as well. Couples may hire a childbirth assistant to give backup support, to interface with hospital staff, and to do odd jobs, freeing the father for just caressing and holding his mate. If you hire a childbirth assistant:

- interview the childbirth assistant to be sure the person is someone with whom both parents get along.
- be sure the assistant is fully supportive of your birth plans.
- find out what she usually does during labor. Is the assistant's role limited to giving labor support, or is she also willing to help out during the early postpartum period?

Noa Ben-Amotz Mitchell, a childbirth assistant who teaches alternative-birth classes and home-birth workshops in Nashville, Tennessee, says, "My role depends on what the couple needs and what the father feels comfortable offering." When she works in hospitals, where the support of a professional is often more needed than at a home or childbearing-center birth, she acts as a consumer advocate in addition to giving hands-on labor support: "I help couples understand the choices that are presented to them and help them make informed decisions."

Cheri, a new mother, recalls: "We wanted a childbirth assistant for a couple of reasons. First, in case we had to transfer to the hospital, I felt it was important to have someone who understood our needs. I didn't want my husband, Martin, to run interference for me through labor. Second, I wanted him at my side the whole time completely focused on me and not to have to leave for anything. Kathy, my childbirth assistant, did lots of odd jobs like keeping the crock pot warm."

Many fathers prefer to be the sole and primary support person with no one else present during labor. However, for other couples, the childbirth assistant can enhance the father's ability to give effective support in the way that is most comfortable for him.

"During one labor," Noa Mitchell recalls, "the husband didn't feel comfortable giving hands-on practical help. While I filled that need based on my experience, the husband was able to relax and trust his instincts without fearing the responsibility of having to give the major support. He provided the emotional support—hugging his mate, whispering encouraging words, being intimate that only a partner can provide."

Choosing Childbirth Classes

Good classes will provide an opportunity to learn about labor and your options regarding birth, air your concerns, and meet other expectant parents who probably share many of your feelings.

When selecting classes, choose carefully. The best classes are usually small—with no more than ten couples. Those held on neutral ground (in a private home or a church, for example) are usually preferable to those sponsored by a hospital. Though many hospital classes are excellent, most do not encourage mothers to learn about alternatives and take an active role in their own health care. Rather than give the parents the information they need to make well-informed decisions, instructors all too frequently prepare the mother to accept hospital policies and medical routines.

Other features of good classes are that they are supportive of breastfeeding and cover information about preventing unnecessary cesarean sections, not merely facts about cesarean surgery.

Finally, good classes should inspire *both* parents' confidence in their ability to handle labor—the mother's confidence in her strength and power and the father's confidence in his ability to give effective labor support, reducing his mate's fear and discomfort.

When my wife and I discovered we were going to have our first child, we signed up for childbirth classes. During the first class, the instructor assumed that all her clients were planning a hospital birth without asking whether some might prefer to give birth in other surroundings. We never went back to that class.

Interview the childbirth educator and find out what he or she teaches. It is important to find out your childbirth educator's opinion about EFM, intravenous feeding, episiotomy, and so on. Many instructors do not teach the disadvantages as well as the advantages of medical intervention during labor; in fact, many don't know this information themselves.

Does your childbirth educator present home, childbearing-center, and hospital birth on equal footing? If you can't find an educator who does this in your area, it may be better to educate yourselves. You can start with the reading list at the end of this book.

Using Guided Imagery to Prepare for Birth and Cope with Labor

In many childbirth classes, the instructor will concentrate on teaching couples various permutations of breathing patterns. While some mothers benefit from breathing methods, I strongly recommend using guided imagery in addition to, or in place of, breathing patterns to cope with contractions.

Guided imagery (sometimes called *visualization*) is a means of translating positive thoughts into dynamic mental pictures or images. You can use it for a number of goals, including reducing tension, fear, and pain; developing confidence in your ability to cope with labor; making better birth plans; and enhancing prenatal bonding and the sense of communication with your unborn child.

Guided imagery has been used for centuries in healing. Today, the method has sparked the enthusiasm of professionals the world over. It is used with great success in a wide variety of fields including medicine, psychotherapy, education, business-management training, stress management, and sports training and competition. It is also tremendously effective for childbirth.

THE BENEFITS OF USING GUIDED IMAGERY
THROUGH THE CHILDBEARING SEASON

Laboring women and childbirth professionals who have used guided imagery through the childbearing season have found the method to have all the following benefits. During pregnancy, guided imagery:

- helps both parents make better birth plans
- promotes deep relaxation of body and mind
- develops the mother's confidence in her ability to give birth safely and positively
- develops the father's confidence in the birth process and in his ability to give effective labor support
- enhances prenatal bonding
- reduces the likelihood of postpartum blues

During labor, guided imagery:

- helps the mother relax
- reduces fear
- reduces pain
- may reduce the length of labor
- reduces the likelihood of complications, including fetal distress and cesarean section
- enhances parent–infant bonding
- helps the parents create a safe, positive birth experience

Childbirth educators, nurses, and physicians who have used guided imagery seem to unanimously agree that it is the most effective way to prepare for birth and cope with labor regardless of whether the mother plans a natural birth or a traditional hospital delivery.

For example, Suzanna May Hilbers, teacher-trainer for

ASPO/Lamaze (the world's largest childbirth-education organization), who has used the method with hundreds of laboring women, told me: "Guided imagery is without doubt the most powerful resource a couple has for reducing the fear and pain of labor."

Emmett Miller, M.D., world pioneer in the field of psychophysiological (mind/body) medicine, agrees. After using guided imagery in his practice with pregnant and laboring women, he told me he has found that the method can reduce the need for pain-relief medication and the need for obstetric intervention, including the use of forceps.

Many women don't realize how effective guided imagery is until they are actually in labor and the laboring mind response has been elicited. For example, one woman told me that at first she didn't like the exercises I taught because they didn't offer the discipline of Lamaze breathing. However, when she was in active labor, the breathing patterns she had learned in childbirth classes and practiced during pregnancy did not reduce her tension and pain, at which point she used the guided-imagery exercises. After a beautiful natural birth, she exclaimed: "I never thought guided imagery would be helpful. But that's what got me through labor!"

For most women, guided imagery is more effective in reducing tension and childbirth pain than patterned breathing. However, the method can be combined with breathing patterns for those who wish to use both.

WHY DOES GUIDED IMAGERY WORK?
Guided imagery is ideally suited to the expectant and laboring mother. The reason the method works so well in reducing fear and pain in labor can be explained in terms of two characteristics of the laboring mind response: greater right-brain-hemisphere orientation and greater openness to suggestion.

Guided imagery is a right-hemisphere process. Since you are more right-hemisphere-oriented during labor, the method is probably more effective in labor than at any other time in your ordinary waking life. According to Dr. Miller, guided imagery translates cognitive information into terms that can activate the right hemisphere and actually help bring about an easier, more fulfilling labor.

Guided imagery also gives you strong positive suggestions at a time when you are wide open to suggestion. To make the method even more effective, you can combine guided imagery with "affirmations," or strong positive statements, such as "I am able to give birth in harmony with nature" and "I trust my body to labor smoothly and efficiently."

Following are two popular and very effective guided-imagery exercises. See the list of suggested reading at the end of this book for books containing more exercises.

Getting in Touch With Your Unborn Child

Of all the guided-imagery exercises I teach for pregnancy, the following exercise is the most popular. After doing this exercise, one mother said, "It gives me a wonderful, reassuring feeling, a sense of inner strength and power, and of knowing that my baby and I are making this passage together." A father said, "I had the peaceful sense of staring into my child's eyes, just sharing love between the two of us."

This exercise can help you enhance prenatal bonding, develop confidence in your ability to give birth normally, make better birth plans, and heighten prenatal intuition.

Both parents can do the exercise. First, go into a quiet room; remove constricting clothing such as belts, shoes, and glasses; and adopt a relaxing position. Either read through the entire exercise first and then do the imagery or have someone read the exercise to you, giving you plenty of time to complete each step before going to the next. This is your time to take an inner journey to a special place: the very center of your pregnancy—the womb.

RADIANT LIGHT

Begin by breathing deeply and rhythmically, in through the nose and out either through the nose or through slightly parted lips—whichever you prefer.

Become aware of your breathing, and as you do, let your breathing become a little deeper, a little slower, without straining or forcing the breath in any way.

Now, imagine that each breath you take in is a soft, golden, radiant light.

You can think of this light any way you want—as

something real, such as life energy, or as something imaginary, such as a metaphor for the breath.

Breathe this radiant light right into the center of your being.

Let each breath you take in fill you more and more with this soft, golden, radiant light.

And let each breath you let out relax you more and more. Each exhalation melts tension away more and more.

Now, *mothers*: imagine that you are able to breathe this soft, golden, radiant light directly into your womb.

With each breath this radiant light fills your womb— the womb that is the center of your pregnancy, the center of all the changes taking place in your body, your emotions, and your mind.

Meanwhile, *fathers*: continue to breathe this radiant light into the very center of your being.

And, as you do, imagine that this light is somehow able to connect you, to link you, with your unborn child.

Now, both mothers and fathers, imagine that your mind, your consciousness, is somehow able to be in the womb with your baby and that you are face to face with your unborn child.

Visualize the baby in any way that feels comfortable to you. You don't have to be concerned with how the baby actually appears at this state of development; just picture the baby in whatever way feels right.

Perhaps you imagine the baby lying head down surrounded by a crystal-clear sea of amniotic fluid in his or her own private universe—perfectly comfortable, secure, . . . at peace.

Enjoy being with your unborn child in this unique way for a little while.

And, as you do, if you find your attention wandering or if irrelevant thoughts come into your mind, gently bring your awareness back to your baby by mentally repeating the word *baby* with each breath you let out.

And let yourself go into an even deeper state of relaxation—of body and mind.

Now, allow the love you feel for your child to well up within you. And, as you do, you may want to talk with your baby. Tell your child anything you want: how you are feeling right now, how much you are looking forward to holding him or her in your arms, how much you love him or her . . . anything you want.

You may even want to ask your baby a question: What do you most need right now? Where would you like to be born? What will you most need during the first week after birth? . . . any question you wish.

Imagine that your baby can answer you—in words, images, or impressions, by painting a picture in your mind's eye.

Don't be surprised if, while doing this exercise, you glimpse the baby's gender or some aspect of the baby's physical characteristics, or get a sense of the baby's personality. This is perfectly normal.

For now, dwell on the love you feel for your unborn child.

And, as you do this, tell yourself: I am able and willing to give my child everything he or she needs to grow and be healthy.

When you are ready to return to your everyday waking life, take a few deep breaths, stretch gently, and open your eyes.

To enhance the bond both parents share with their unborn child, while doing this exercise, focus on the love you and your child share.

To develop confidence in your ability to give birth normally, take a mental tour of the womb. Then express gratitude for the miracle that has already taken place—the creation of your child. Remind yourself that by the time labor begins, most of the hard work—the creation of a baby—is already over. By thinking this you are not minimizing the hard work of labor, but becoming aware of the awesome creative miracle your body has already performed.

To make better birth plans, ask the baby, "Where would you like to be born?" and allow your mind to remain open for a possible "answer." It is not necessary to believe your child actually answers the question. You can think of the baby's answer as a metaphor for your own inner thoughts.

In answer to your question, you may imagine a birth place suffused with peace and love, or you may receive no impression, in which case you will still have opened your mind to considering the birth place from the baby's point of view. In any event, few self-respecting fetuses—metaphorical or real—are likely to respond, "I'd like to be yanked out in a stainless-steel delivery room under bright lights."

To enhance your intuition, ask the baby a question as discussed above and allow your mind to be open to "receiving" an answer. Possible questions are: What do I most need to do now to prepare for a safe, positive birth? What will you most need during the first few weeks after birth? and so on.

This exercise is a way of bypassing your logical mind and getting in touch with your own inner resources. Both are necessary for a rich, full childbirth experience.

THE OPENING FLOWER

Many women find this exercise effective for coping with contractions and hastening labor's progress. The opening flower is an ideal metaphor for the dilating cervix during the first stage and the opening birth canal during the second. No image better captures the qualitiesof warmth, beauty, softness, moisture, fragrance, andopening.

During contractions, imagine a blossoming flower. Choose any flower at all—a rose, lily, a water lily—as long as it is beautiful. Then imagine the flower opening slowly, petal by petal, opening . . . opening . . . opening . . . until it is fully in blossom.

You can add as many details to this exercise as you want, such as imagining the shape of the petals, their delicate or bold shading, dewdrops on the flower, its fragrance, or the sun's rays coaxing the flower to open.

You can also vary the exercise by imagining that you are in a beautiful garden surrounded by hundreds of flowers. You can take a mental journey in the garden and choose the most beautiful flower of all, then imagine that flower blossoming, petal by petal.

Linda, a mother who used guided imagery, recalls: "Visualizations and relaxation were an important part of my prenatal care. The visualization of an opening flower is used to help enhance the opening of the cervix during labor. My husband, being a horticulturalist, suggested the image of a hibiscus. It was the biggest flower we could think of! I made a tape of the visualizations so I could listen to it whenever I chose."

After a beautiful natural birth at home, Linda says: "My husband, Bill, my son, Ryan, and I all gazed adoringly at this new baby and I knew a joy more complete than any I had ever known before. . . . The placenta has a special place in our garden, nourishing the hibiscus plants my husband gave me during my pregnancy. When the baby was one week old the hibiscus bloomed. The flower was beautiful and huge, just like in my visualization . . . a wonderful symbol of what we had planned and hoped for and at last experienced."

The Lamaze Method

The Lamaze method, also called the "psychoprophylactic" method, was originally introduced by French obstetrician Dr. Ferdinand Lamaze. This method provides knowledge of the anatomy and physiology of labor to help the expectant mother overcome fear, relaxation practice to diminish tension and pain during contractions, and breathing patterns to be used as an aid to relaxation or as a distraction during contractions. Today, however, the term "Lamaze classes" has come to describe a wide variety of childbirth classes, some having almost nothing in common with one another.

Most Lamaze instructors teach patterned breathing. Hundreds of Lamaze childbirth educators have also learned about the benefits of guided imagery and are teaching this in place of, or in addition to, the breathing.

Childbirth educators teach a wide variety of breathing patterns to help the laboring woman relax and cope with contractions and to distract her from the pain. These include:

- *slow breathing,* to be used when contractions are mild
- *accelerated or light breathing,* to be used when contractions are more difficult
- *pant-blow* breathing, to be used when contractions are at their most difficult.

Breathing patterns help many laboring women reduce the fear and pain of labor. However, not all women find patterned breathing helpful in reducing tension or pain. In addition, it can be tiring, particularly during a long labor.

I don't teach breathing patterns for a number of reasons. For many mothers, these patterns interfere with a spontaneous response to labor and can actually impede labor's progress. Also, fathers frequently become so involved in coaching their mates with patterned breathing that they lose sight of what are often more effective means of labor support, such as whispering encouraging words or hugging the laboring woman.

However, since patterned breathing does help some laboring women, you may want to learn the method. I recommend learning about using guided imagery as well and first trying that method. Think of the breathing patterns as backup, using them *when and if* you find the need.

As I mentioned earlier, patterned breathing and guided imagery can be combined quite effectively. For example, you can use the "Opening Flower" or other imagery exercises while breathing deeply and rhythmically. Or you can do the following Radiant Breath imagery during contractions.

RADIANT BREATH

Imagine that with each breath you take in, you are breathing in a soft, golden, radiant light.

Imagine that this light is filling your body.

Now, direct the radiant light to any part of the body that is tense or uncomfortable and imagine the tension or discomfort being massaged away by a million invisible fingers of radiant light.

Meanwhile, imagine that each breath you let out melts tension away, more and more.

AFTER THE BIRTH

A colleague once told me that tales of women who give birth only to return to work immediately afterward are fictional. Women can't really do that, she claimed. But she's wrong: that's just what my wife did after the birth of our third child, Jonathan. Within an hour, she was up cooking a meal, while I, on the other hand, was so exhausted I could barely walk!

As long as there are no medical complications, you can be up and about as soon as you want after birth. The father can help you the first time you get out of bed in case you feel dizzy, lightheaded, weak in the knees, or faint. However, you will require plenty of rest during the early postpartum period—even if you are one of those unusual women like Jan who insists on being active immediately after giving birth. (Jan finally did sit down at the insistence of our midwife!) Limit your activities to taking care of yourself and your baby for the first week or so after birth.

Plan to have help around the home. The life-altering era after the birth of your baby is no time to try to be self-sufficient. It is quite appropriate to depend on your family and perhaps friends for a few days or longer.

The father can take charge of all household responsibilities, but he should not try to do all the work himself. I suggest that he delegate most of the work to family members, friends, or, perhaps, hired help. He, too, needs time to adjust to his new baby, and he also will probably need rest.

I'll never forget how much it meant to us when my own mother helped Jan and me after our second son, Paul, was born. She stayed with us for a few days, cooked, cleaned, shopped, and even took little trips with our son Carl, who was two years old at the time.

"My mother and my husband's mother came to our home from time to time to clean up and cook and friends brought food," recalls Ann of the days after her baby was born. "This gave me time to rest and nurse my daughter, who wanted to nurse constantly."

One couple, Jean and Tony, belong to a church that sends meals to parents' homes for two weeks after birth—a great gift for the new family. You may want to let relatives know you would appreciate a home-cooked meal or other help as a baby gift.

Family members and friends should focus on the new parents' needs and helping out at home rather than assuming baby-care responsibilities. Of course, grandparents will find it irresistible to spend some time cuddling the baby. And you can hardly expect anyone to do housework without being allowed to enjoy the best part! But, for the most part, you should take on the role of baby care and learn to trust your own ability—even though you may feel awkward or want to rely on others at first.

Be sure the persons who are helping out are supportive of your chosen method of childbirth, breastfeeding, and whatever aspects of parenting are important to you. It does little good to have relatives helping out who are constantly criticizing your parenting style.

Try to limit visitors. Even helpful visitors can be exhausting for the new family. However, as in most everything in childbearing, let how you feel physically and emotionally be your guide.

Paternity Leave

Martin, a new father, remained home for a week after the birth of his child. His paternity leave was unpaid. "I can't imagine how I would have done it if I hadn't had him home!" exclaims his wife, Cheri. "I have one flat and one inverted nipple and had some problems breastfeeding. We didn't know anyone who had breastfed, but Martin was very supportive. In the middle of the night when I was exhausted and had absolutely no patience, he was able to be there for me when I needed him."

I strongly urge every new father—regardless of where the birth takes place—to take a week to be with his unfolding family and help out around the home. Though most men won't be paid for the time off work, they'll find the benefits of taking paternity leave outweigh the financial loss. The father will find it easier to adjust to his new fathering role if he is with his family without interruption for a few days. He can help out with cooking, cleaning, doing the laundry, and other chores and give the mother much-needed emotional support. And as a final benefit, he can rest.

"I stayed in bed for most of the first week after birth, getting up just to shower and change diapers," Maryann recalls. "Mark did the cooking and cleaning. When I wanted to take a nap, he'd take the baby and sleep with her on the couch until she wanted to nurse."

In my opinion, the father should take paternity leave whether or not the parents have others to help out around the home or plan to hire professional help. Nothing substitutes for the father's presence. Though there may be others to meet the mother's practical needs, the father is still needed to cope with the deeply emotional adjustments and realities of shared parenthood.

The Postpartum Assistant

In many areas, professional postpartum assistants are available to new families. Such assistants now often replace the mother or grandmother who traditionally helped the new mother through the first few days after the birth a few generations ago.

Postpartum assistants do a wide variety of jobs, from house-cleaning and cooking to giving breastfeeding help. Many take vital signs (temperature, pulse, and respiration), examine the mother to ensure she is recovering properly, and answer basic health questions.

The services of these professionals are becoming increasingly widespread as more and more families opt for early discharge from hospitals or plan to give birth at home or in childbearing centers. To locate one in your area, phone a local La Leche League group for a listing of childbirth educators in your area, contact a hospital maternity unit, or check the ads in a local parenting publication.

Important Phone Numbers

Phone numbers of persons who can answer questions about breastfeeding and give you other health information should be available at your fingertips after the baby is born.

For a breastfeeding specialist, get the telephone number of a lactation consultant, a local nursing mother's information service, or a La Leche League group. Lactation consultants are highly trained professionals who charge for their services. Local nursing mother's information services are available through many childbirth-education organizations. A nursing counselor may be able to talk with you on the phone and perhaps even visit your home at no charge, and some local maternity units are also willing to answer questions over the phone.

A local childbirth educator should be able to give you telephone numbers. (La Leche League International [LLLI] is a worldwide organization that provides information in most cities in the United States. If you can't find a local La Leche League group listed in your phone directory, call the national office for a referral. See Resources.) Most childbirth educators are willing to answer questions about baby care and maternal health issues. If you have taken childbirth classes, have your childbirth educator's telephone number handy.

LOOKING AHEAD

The chapters ahead will give you information about midwifery care and each of the major methods of alternative birth. Each method will require some additional preparation. (For example, the parents who choose home birth should select a backup hospital in case a transfer is needed.) Choosing your method of childbirth to meet your individual needs and preparing carefully are giant steps toward creating the safe, rewarding childbirth experience you, your mate, and your child deserve.

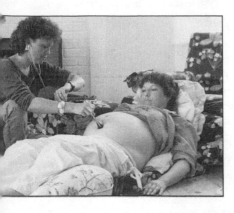

CHAPTER 4

Midwifery Care

DONNA AND KARL, BOTH CLINI-cal psychologists in New Jersey, were so committed to midwifery care that it was either a midwife or no attendant at all. In Donna's words: "I didn't want to relinquish control over one of the most intensely personal events in Karl's and my life. We intended to birth our baby together with people who respected our needs and intelligence." During labor, with her husband and midwife to support her, Donna recalls "feeling encircled with love and safety."

Thousand of parents have had similar experiences. Midwives are becoming the choice caregivers for a growing number of mothers who have discovered that they offer safe, personal obstetrical care that in many ways is superior to the care offered by most physicians.

Throughout most of history, midwives have played a prominent role in the lives of childbearing families. "It is the oldest honorable profession," says Janet Tipton, a midwife in East Texas. They were respected and honored the world over. However, the past couple of centuries brought dramatic changes. Midwifery care fell into disrepute in Europe and was virtually eradicated in the United States. Today, that trend is being reversed. Midwives are again rising in popularity. The number of hospital births attended by midwives has increased a full five times from 1975 to 1987 and continues to grow. The number of midwife-attended home births is seeing a similar jump.

Midwifery is being reborn.

THE DEMISE AND REBIRTH OF MIDWIFERY CARE

The near demise of the world's most ancient health profession is one of the strangest and darkest chapters in childbirth history.

As early as the eighteenth century, "male midwives" (an old name for doctors who provided obstetric care) became fashionable. Despite initial cultural resistance, women—particularly middle- and upper-class women—came to prefer the male midwives because they appeared to have more overall medical knowledge. Initially, the choice was the childbearing women's. However, physicians in Europe and America began to wage a bitter campaign to defame and devalue traditional midwives.

At the same time, midwives, working more or less independently of one another, lacked organization, leadership, and educational programs (though there were still a few midwifery schools dating from the sixteenth century). As a result, though experience and skills varied from one midwife to another, the practice of many midwives became outdated while the medical profession continued to advance. In addition, lack of licensure requirements and formal supervision kept midwives from being officially recognized as part of the health-care system.

Physicians brought both great advances and dire perils to childbirth. On the positive side, they made midwifery a science, the forerunner of obstetrics. Doctors established programs of education, published books, and developed technological interventions to assist women in childbirth when nature failed.

However, as doctors replaced the midwives, a pattern that is only beginning to be reversed developed. Physicians overused interventive methods, sometimes causing illness and death. Under the physician's care, birth became less of a social event shared by the family. And worse, doctors introduced the most gruesome chapter in the history of childbirth: puerperal fever. During the nineteenth century, puerperal or "childbed" fever, a severe, often fatal, infection, reached epidemic proportions, killing thousands of new mothers. This terrible tragedy was created by doctors and nurses who failed to wash their hands after examining cadavers or ill patients before doing vaginal exams. The infection was also carried from one mother to another by the doctors and nurses. Most women who gave birth at home—or even on the hospital steps and corridors on their way to the maternity wards—were spared. The infection raged until the latter part of the nineteenth century, when antiseptic hand-washing became standard practice.

Nowhere on earth did midwives come as close to being eradicated as in the United States. Midwives were among the first people to settle the colonies, and by the turn of the twentieth century, they were still delivering about half the babies born. Yet by 1935, midwives were delivering only about 12 percent of babies. The trend toward doctor-managed labor continued until the 1970s, when physicians were delivering well over 95 percent and probably closer to 100 percent, of all babies born.

While midwives are still fighting for recognition in the United States, they hold a far higher status in other developed countries. For example, whereas under 5 percent of births are attended by midwives in the United States, nearly three-quarters of births are attended by midwives in Great Britain. Midwives are respected in nations with far lower infant-mortality rates than that of the United States, such as the Netherlands, Denmark, and Japan where these health professionals attend somewhere between 60 and 80 percent of all births.

WHAT IS A MIDWIFE?

A midwife is a person who gives prenatal care, delivers babies, gives postpartum care, provides normal newborn care, and, in some cases, provides well-woman care.

Midwife Means *With Woman*

Midwives are fond of quoting the literal meaning of their title—from the Anglo-Saxon *mid,* "with," and *wif,* "woman." The expression "*midwife* means 'with woman'" is becoming popular in childbirth circles. I've seen it on bumper stickers, cloth tote bags, and T-shirts. It emphasizes the midwife's commitment to working with the mother, or as some put it, "to serving the childbearing woman."

In 1955, the American College of Nurse-Midwives (ACNM) was established to certify members of their profession. Gradually, nurse-midwives have become nationally recognized health professionals. They have also formed state, regional, and national networks to promote alternative birth and to work toward the legalization of their practice. In 1982, the Midwives Alliance of North America (MANA) was founded to improve communication among all midwives and to establish guidelines for basic competency and safety. MANA is a member of the International Confederation of Midwives, which sets standards for the practice of midwifery worldwide.

Both men and women practice midwifery. In 1988, however, less than one hundred of the four thousand certified nurse-midwives who practiced in the United States were men. Yet, more men are becoming interested in the profession as stereotypes identifying nursing and midwifery as "women's work" crumble.

THE QUALITIES OF A GOOD MIDWIFE

More important than gender are the qualities that distinguish a good midwife. Most childbirth professionals agree that the ideal midwife should have a thorough background in the anatomy and physiology of pregnancy and labor, be able to recognize complications, work in close collaboration with a backup physician and hospital should a transfer be necessary, and be flexible enough to meet the parents' individual goals. They should also have a nonjudgmental approach and have, as one physician put it, "a lot of love in the heart."

Though *midwife* and *midwifery* refer to a specific health profession, these terms also have a broader meaning. Some physicians and midwives think of midwifery as noninterventive obstetric care *regardless of who provides that care*. As one family physician put it: "I think of midwifery as a style of practice and I'm honored to have my clients think of me as a midwife." In this sense of the term, a physician, naturopath, or chiropractor, as well as a midwife, can practice midwifery.

Midwives practice in homes, childbearing centers, and hospitals throughout the world. The places where they practice vary with the regulations of different areas and with the individual midwife's preference.

Some midwives are acknowledged, recognized, and respected by the government in the place they reside; others are not. All, however, perform a vital service for childbearing families.

TYPES OF MIDWIVES

Several types of midwives of varying backgrounds give prenatal care and attend births.

A *certified nurse-midwife* or *CNM* (often called *nurse-midwife*) is a person educated in both nursing and midwifery who possesses evidence of certification according to the requirements of the American College of Nurse-Midwives (ACNM).

A *direct-entry midwife* is often called *midwife, independent midwife,* in some states *certified* or *licensed lay midwife, traditional midwife,* or *empirical midwife.* In Europe, a direct-entry midwife is one who has been trained in midwifery school with or without prior training in nursing. In the United States, this term is often used to refer to a midwife who has entered the profession through apprenticeship training, through midwifery schooling, from a background of nursing practice, or a combination. *Direct-entry midwife* is sometimes also used as a synonym for *lay midwife,* though the former is becoming the preferred term.

A *lay midwife* is one who has entered the profession through apprenticeship with an experienced midwife or physician, through midwifery schooling, or a combination of both. These midwives have varying levels of skill and experience. In some states, midwives who are not CNMs are licensed to practice and are regulated by a governing board of health professionals.

A *granny midwife* is a person who acts as a lay midwife helping neighboring women give birth. Granny midwives are most common in the rural South, where they serve a predominantly black population. Most are not formally educated and have no medical background, though they may work closely with public health or medical professionals. Granny midwives are becoming less and less common.

A *nurse-midwife* is a nurse who acts as a midwife attending births but is not certified.

MIDWIVES AND THEIR TRAINING

Two major types of midwives practice in the United States today: certified nurse-midwives and direct-entry midwives.

The Certified Nurse-Midwife (CNM)

A certified nurse-midwife is educated in both nursing and midwifery. Being a Registered Nurse is a prerequisite for nurse-midwifery education. CNMs receive their practical hands-on experience in a variety of settings including hospitals, clinics, birth centers, and home-birth practices. On completion of the educational program, the midwife receives evidence of certification from the American College of Certified Nurse-Midwives (ACNM), the professional organization for nurse-midwives.

CNMs are well-trained. Having received much clinical experience in large teaching hospitals, they are experienced in giving prenatal care, assisting during childbirth, and recognizing complications. They are also educated in well-woman gynecology and newborn care.

One of my acquaintances, Mary Ellen Doherty, CNM, received her certification through the Nurse-Midwifery Program at the University of Medicine and Dentistry in New Jersey. After practicing in Emerson Hospital in Concord, Massachusetts for a few years, she and two other nurse-midwives opened a private practice, Concord Nurse-Midwifery Associates. The midwives work in collaboration with three backup physicians in case of complications.

Another CNM, Vicky Wolfrum of South Bay Family Care in San Pedro, California, has a unique background. She was originally trained in Switzerland through apprenticeship. She became a registered nurse and began to work in California, a state where lay midwifery is illegal. "You can't keep the clients' best interest at heart if you're worried about breaking the law," she says. So she became a CNM and now attends both home and childbearing-center births.

CNMs are *required* to work in a collaborative relationship with a physician and to have physician backup.

Other Midwives

Internationally, the term *direct entry midwife* refers to a person who has completed formal education in midwifery and is licensed or certified to practice in his or her state or province. In the United States, however, this term is often used to refer to all midwives other than CNMs. Usually this means midwives who have entered the profession "directly," without first having become a nurse. However, some nurses have also trained to become midwives without becoming CNMs.

In some states, such as Washington and Arizona, formal schooling is required for midwives; therefore the word *lay* is inappropriate and is resented by midwives. In other states such as New Hampshire, *lay* is the officially accepted term.

In this chapter, I use the term *direct-entry midwife* to refer to all midwives who are not CNMs, nurses or otherwise. (Midwives are by no means in accord about what they should be called. During a lunch with a group of midwives who all had similar training, I received no less than six different responses from seven women when I asked about the proper name of their profession. One said she thought of herself as an *empirical midwife*; another preferred the term *practical midwife*; a third and fourth liked the term *traditional midwife*; a fifth called herself a *lay midwife*; a sixth, who was licensed to practice in New Hampshire, called herself a *licensed midwife*; and the seventh preferred *direct-entry midwife*. After the lunch, I told another midwife about all these terms. She said: "I don't like any of them. I call myself an 'independent midwife.'")

The background and training of direct-entry midwives can be as varied as their names. Many are trained through apprenticeship, in midwifery school, or through a combination of the two.

I know several former maternity nurses who have decided to become midwives. Many have had extensive experience and witnessed thousands of births before deciding to attend births at home. For example, Lisa Jensen, a midwife practicing in Lyman, New Hampshire, is a registered nurse who was trained in midwifery through apprenticeship. Now she is in a community-based nurse-midwifery program working toward becoming a CNM.

A few midwives are empirically trained; that is, they began attending births with no background in the field. For example, CharLynn Daughtry, who runs the Labor of Love Childbirth Center in Lakeland, Florida, was empirically trained through self-study and attending births on her own. "I would tell parents that I was not a midwife," CharLynn recalls, "but I would offer them the experience I had at no charge." She trained this way for five years and is now licensed by the state of Florida.

Another midwife, Joan Remington, founder of the Northern Arizona School of Midwifery, attended her first birth in 1975. "The mother was planning to give birth at home, unattended," she recalls. "Two of us who had given birth previously planned to be with her. The baby was born easily, and mother and baby were perfectly healthy. When I suctioned mucus from the baby's mouth and cut the cord, I realized that birth was such a significant event that I had to do more than just attend, believing all would be well. If a problem did develop, I had no skills to handle it. So, I decided I would go and get training." Today Joan is a licensed midwife working with a partner, Mary Ann Baul, in Womancare Midwifery Associates in Flagstaff, Arizona. They have attended 450 births since 1982 with no infant mortalities.

Direct-entry midwives have varied degrees of skill and experience. They range from highly skilled, qualified, experienced caregivers to persons who claim to be midwives after having observed one or two births.

Inadequate training is more likely if the midwife's experience comes solely through attending home births as an apprentice. Unless she is in a major city apprenticing for an unusually busy midwife, she would have to spend many years in training to be highly experienced.

Midwifery Schools

The Netherlands is a country with one of the world's lowest infant-mortality rates. Midwives there train in a midwifery school for three years. They observe and participate in hundreds of births and witness complications as well as normal births. Their midwifery system is impressive.

During the mother's labor, Dutch midwives work with "home helpers" who act as birth assistants. The home helper is trained to assist the midwife during labor and to help the mother and infant for ten days after birth. Like postpartum assistants in the United States, the home helper does light housekeeping and cooking in addition to caring for the mother and baby.

Dutch midwives are not nurses. They are independent professionals who have no affiliation with hospitals, nurses, or physicians. They do not follow the rules and protocol of other professionals overseeing their activities, but rely on their own professional protocol.

Many direct-entry midwives envision themselves as the American counterparts of the Dutch midwife. Several midwifery schools such as the Northern Arizona School of Midwifery and the Seattle Midwifery School provide training in midwifery that includes many areas of health care, skill, and study that overlap a nursing curriculum.

There are differences between the Dutch midwife and her American counterpart, however. The Dutch midwife is part of an entire nationwide system of medical care. She is acknowledged, recognized, respected as an integral part of the health-care system. In the eyes of everyone, she is a professional. She is able to provide maternity care in hospitals as well as at home. In striking contrast, in 1990, the U.S. direct-entry midwife could not officially provide health care in hospitals (though direct-entry midwives are now seeking hospital privileges). In most states, the medical establishment does not recognize the direct-entry midwife as a professional.

Some midwifery schools offer thorough instruction for direct-entry midwives. For example, the Seattle Midwifery School, founded in 1978, combines classroom instruction and clinical training with community-based practicing midwives. Relying on European standards for academic content and clinical experience for direct-entry midwifery programs, the school was the first to successfully pilot comprehensive, professional midwifery training leading to state licensure.

Another similar school, the Northern Arizona School of Midwivery in Flagstaff, requires 920 hours of clinical experience in addition to rigorous academic requirements. The school also requires that midwifery students attend and participate in 100 prenatal visits, 100 newborn exams, 100 postpartum exams, and 100 births.

Two very busy childbearing centers now offer midwifery training in El Paso: Maternidad La Luz and Casa da Nacamiento. Karen Miller, acting director of Maternidad La Luz, justifiably refers to El Paso as the "Mecca of Midwifery training." No other location in the U.S. offers so much experience in such a short time. Both schools provide clinical experience at prenatal exams and during labor on site. Students who complete the training then continue apprenticing with other midwives.

Unfortunately, these schools lack ongoing affiliation agreements with hospitals and most students' experience is limited to home and childbearing center birth. Hopefully, this will change as direct-entry midwives become more widely accepted and officially recognized.

The Midwife's View of Birth

Most midwives—CNMs as well as direct-entry midwives—view birth as a normal, natural process. The majority are committed to providing noninterventive maternity care.

"I had my first baby overseas with nurse-midwives and they were wonderful," says Mary Hammond-Tooke, CNM, of the Maternity Center in Bethesda, Maryland, who attends both home and childbearing-center births. "When I came back to the U.S., I had the misconception that I would receive better care since America is so advanced in so many other areas. But during my next labor, I was appalled at the care I received. The nurses who attended me during labor were not at all helpful. They kept pushing drugs. They didn't understand natural childbirth. After the baby was born, I wasn't allowed to nurse right away. They were so unsupportive of breastfeeding that if I hadn't breastfed the first baby, I would never have breastfed. I decided to become a midwife and help mothers do it differently."

Though most midwives embrace a philosophy of noninterventive care, practice styles vary from one practitioner to another. I've observed midwives who cut episiotomies on every first-time mother and who use electronic fetal monitoring routinely. However, the majority of midwives I've seen at birth help the mother give birth the way the mother chooses without unnecessary intervention.

There is some disagreement about which midwives provide better care: CNMs or direct-entry midwives. Some certified nurse-midwives feel that one can't acquire adequate obstetric skills without first becoming a nurse. On the other hand, some direct-entry midwives claim that a nurse has too much of a medical focus to be a good midwife. In my opinion, whether or not a midwife is a nurse is unimportant providing he or she is skilled and highly experienced.

Physicians and Midwives—the Difference

Though midwives are trained to recognize complications and handle emergencies, midwifery is the only health profession concerned primarily with a normal, natural event and not an affliction or a disease. As a general rule, midwives have a more natural, less interventive approach to childbirth than do physicians.

Bear in mind, however, that this is only a generality. Many obstetricians and family physicians today work with the heart of a midwife, while some midwives work with too-clinical hands.

One would think that obstetricians, with their more advanced education and broader experience, offer better care than midwives. There is certainly no question that obstetricians are better trained to handle complications. However, studies suggest that midwives may be better trained to provide safe obstetrical care during essentially normal pregnancies and labors.

In some ways, the midwife's training may actually be superior to the physician's. Many midwives have skills most obstetricians do not. For example, the majority of midwives know how to protect a woman from tearing by applying warm compresses, doing perineal massage, and gently manipulating the perineum over the baby's head. Peculiar as it may seem, most physicians have not learned these basic skills and most will cut episiotomies instead.

A few obstetricians are beginning to learn skills from home-birth midwives. For example, at a midwifery conference in Baltimore, Maryland, where I was conducting a workshop, two obstetricians had registered to learn skills from a lay-trained midwife.

One important difference between the midwife's and the obstetrician's training is that the midwife has attended many labors from beginning to end. In striking contrast, many physicians have never observed a single labor all the way through: *labor experience is a missing ingredient in established obstetric training.* In hospitals, nurses, not physicians, take care of laboring women unless there are medical complications requiring the obstetrician's expertise. Physicians are expected to learn about labor from studying textbooks and graphs and from the few minutes they spend with laboring women. In my opinion, this is like learning to fish on dry land.

"You can't learn about labor like that!" exclaims one physician, outraged at the quality of medical education in obstetrics. "Without listening to every contraction, being right there with a woman, you can't really know labor. You have to be with a woman throughout her labor: ten, twenty-four, thirty-six hours, however long it takes—until the baby is born."

ADVANTAGES OF MIDWIFERY CARE

Pioneer obstetrician Richard B. Stewart, founder of the Douglas Birthing Center in Douglasville, Georgia, says: "I firmly believe that the best kind of birth a woman can have is to be attended by a trained midwife, or a doctor who practices like a midwife."

Parents opt to have a midwife attend their birth at home, in a childbearing center, or in a hospital for any or all of the following advantages.

Most midwives are committed to giving noninterventive health care through the childbearing season. The mother who chooses a midwife has a greatly reduced chance of having intervention such as electronic fetal monitoring, intravenous feeding, an episiotomy, a cesarean section, and so forth. As Lynn, a California mother, put it: "I trusted by body's ability to give birth naturally and didn't want a lot of unnecessary medical intervention. So I chose a midwife."

Most midwives spend much more time with clients than physicians do. Most of my midwifery acquaintances allot at least thirty minutes for each prenatal visit and often an hour or more for the first visit, to develop a rapport with the client and better meet her needs.

The midwife remains with the mother throughout labor, or for a significant portion of her labor, providing continuity of care. As I've discussed, most obstetricians, by contrast, come in at the last minute to deliver the baby. Again, continuous individual support enables many women to labor more efficiently and feel more secure.

Midwives who attend home or childbearing-center births will often accompany the mother if she must be transferred to the hospital. There, the midwife continues to provide support and, in some hospitals, may also provide medical care.

The mother attended by a midwife has a significantly reduced chance of having an unnecessary cesarean section. Carol, a mother in Florida, says: "My cervix was so slow to dilate that my gynecologist told me that I would have had a cesarean section had I been in the hospital. However, I had chosen a midwife who stayed with me and encouraged me to give birth naturally."

This mother is not alone. Numerous studies have shown that the cesarean rate among midwifery clients is a fraction of that of women attended by obstetricians.

Midwives support family-centered care. Most midwives view the father as an intrinsic part of the childbearing experience. Family participation is encouraged if the couple desires.

Midwives provide emotional support as well as physical care throughout labor. Most midwives help the mother deal with her feelings about becoming a parent and her fears about childbirth and give her encouragement. This boosts the mother's confidence and often assists her to labor more smoothly.

Midwives support the parents' individual goals. Most midwives encourage parents to actively participate in their birth experience.

Tom, a father in Florida, says he and his wife found their midwife far more committed to helping them with their last four births than was the physician who had provided care during their first birth. "Our first birth was with a doctor," Tom recalls. "He was a wonderful man, but only showed up to deliver the baby. He expected us to do everything his way. The midwife was willing to help us give birth the way we wanted and have the baby in the place we felt most comfortable, which was in our home."

Maggie, a mother of two in Anderson, Indiana, says: "I wasn't happy with my physician. He didn't seem to be concerned about my needs." She switched to a midwife who was so committed to giving personal care that it changed Maggie's outlook on childbirth. "When I first became pregnant," she recalls, "I wanted a hospital birth with medication, but after talking with my midwife, I felt totally at ease about giving birth naturally."

The mother is able to be attended by a woman. Some women choose midwives so that they can receive care from an empathetic woman during labor. Among some ethnic groups, it is unacceptable to have a pelvic examination done by a man. Other women may simply feel more comfortable being attended by a female midwife, particularly one who has given birth herself. A mother in central Florida says: "One reason I chose a midwife was because I felt that a woman who has given birth could better understand and identify with me." This is not true for all women, but if you also feel more comfortable with a woman, trust your instincts and choose one.

Midwives provide care at a cost usually significantly lower than that of obstetricians. Occasionally, however, midwifery care is overly expensive, because in some areas financial arrangements must be made with the backup physician. For example, in California, nurse-midwives work under the supervision of a physician. Should the parents sue for malpractice, it is the physician, not the midwife, who is responsible, unjust as this may be. Accordingly, the cost of midwifery is elevated to pay the physician's malpractice insurance.

BENEFITS OF MIDWIFERY CARE

The following are advantages associated with midwifery care. Bear in mind, however, that the care midwives provide and their attitudes about childbirth vary from one practitioner to another.

- safe, personalized health care throughout the child-bearing season
- noninterventive maternity care
- continuous emotional support through labor
- reduced chance of a cesarean section
- support of the mother's and father's individual goals
- reduced cost in comparison to that of an obstetrician's care

---

WHO HAS MIDWIFERY CARE?

All mothers—low- and high-risk—can benefit from skilled, experienced midwifery care.

For *home and childbearing-center births,* all responsible midwives screen mothers prenatally for complications. Most recommend that their clients also visit a physician to be checked out for conditions that may pose complications during pregnancy or labor. Women who have preeclampsia, kidney disease, heart disease, severe anemia, hypertension, diabetes, abnormal presentations, multiple gestations, placenta previa, pre- or postmature labor, or other complications are usually referred to a physician.

In hospitals, midwives usually provide health care only to the low-risk mothers. However, there are exceptions. For instance, in New York City's North Central Bronx Hospital, where the population is predominantly high-risk, 100 percent of clients receive midwifery care and 80 percent of births are done by midwives. If there are medical complications, a physician may also give health care, but the midwife still remains actively involved.

The often-quoted studies about the safety of midwifery care in inner-city hospitals and rural areas has given many people the impression that midwives provide care for a primarily indigent population. This misconception leads some to assume that midwives provide second-class care. Neither assumption is accurate.

Midwives provide care for mothers of all socioeconomic backgrounds. In fact, surveys have shown that at least 25 percent of CNMs work in private-practice offices with middle- to upper-income clients.

For example, Alice Bailes, CNM of Birthcare and Women's Health in Alexandria, Virginia, attends mothers of all backgrounds from the very upper class to the indigent. Committed to helping women have safe births in the manner they choose, she has even attended a birth in a yurt (an eight-sided Tibetan sod house).

Unfortunately, however, some people still have funny ideas about midwives. When they think of a midwife, the image of some back-country yahoo pops into mind. They don't realize that midwives are bona fide health professionals. Many parents and professionals don't know that many so-called lay midwives may actually be well-trained professionals.

More mothers would opt for midwifery care if they were educated about the safety of this care and about what midwives offer. As one midwife put it: "We have a large number of uneducated consumers that come into nurse-midwifery by chance, not by seeking it. Once they are aware, they love it. We would have a larger clientele if people were more aware of what exactly nurse-midwifery was."

CHOOSING A MIDWIFE

Both certified nurse-midwives and direct-entry midwives practice in every state in the United States. However, in states where direct-entry midwifery has not yet been legalized, midwives who will attend a home birth are not always easy to find. In fact, they remind me of the early persecuted Christians who lived in the catacombs. As Maggie, a mother from Indiana, a state where lay midwifery was illegal as of 1990, says, "After much searching, a CNM gave me the phone number of a lay midwife who would have been prosecuted had she been caught practicing."

Choosing a caregiver has already been discussed in Chapter Three. In addition to the steps outlined in that chapter, keep the following in mind.

Ask about the midwife's background. Where was she trained? How many births has she attended? Midwives vary tremendously in their skill and experience. This is particularly so of those who are not licensed or certified. As Mary Hammond-Tooke of the Maternity Center in Bethesda, Maryland, puts it: "A lay midwife can include everyone from a woman who has watched a couple of births and thinks there is nothing to helping mothers through labor to someone who is highly trained, highly skilled, and very experienced." Though most midwives are highly skilled, some have little experience. Some even train on the job without any background or apprenticeship with more experienced practitioners. The importance of choosing a skilled, experienced midwife cannot be overemphasized.

Find out about your midwife's backup and meet the backup physician. Everyone planning to give birth at home or in a birth center should have a backup physician and hospital in case a last-minute transfer is necessary.

Find out the midwife's philosophy of birth and whether or not it agrees with yours. Midwives differ greatly in their approach. Not all midwives provide noninterventive care; on the other hand, some midwives won't take any action that may be interventive even when necessary.

Find out whether your midwife will continue to provide obstetrical care and/or emotional support if you must be transferred from home or childbearing center to the hospital. Whether or not the midwife remains with the mother throughout her hospital stay depends largely on her relationship with a backup physician and hospital. In some areas, hospitals and backup physicians are not as supportive of midwives as they are in others, and your midwife may not be able to remain with you through no fault of her own.

THE SAFETY OF MIDWIFERY CARE

Medical research has proven that for essentially normal, healthy pregnancies and labors, midwifery care is just as safe as that provided by a physician. Research has shown that midwives working in collaboration with a physician are also safe health-care providers for high-risk mothers. Midwifery care is safe under the following conditions.

- The midwife is well-trained and experienced.
- The midwife works with a physician or has physician backup to handle complications during pregnancy and labor.
- The midwife who is not practicing in a hospital has adequate medical equipment and supplies, including oxygen and infant-resuscitation equipment.
- The midwife who attends childbearing-center and home births has adequate backup at a nearby hospital.

What Medical Studies Show

Medical studies of midwifery care the world over have revealed impressive results. Research has repeatedly proven that well-trained midwives (both direct-entry and certified nurse-midwives) have outstanding health statistics in home, childbearing-center, and hospital settings. Consider these facts.

A higher percentage of midwive-assisted births is associated with decreased infant mortality. As of 1988, the United States, with its large portion of doctor-handled births, has one of the highest infant-mortality rates in the Western world. Among industrialized nations, it ranks a poor nineteenth in the prevention of infant mortality. In Sweden, the country that ranks second in the prevention of infant mortality, nearly all mothers—even those with medical problems requiring the help of a physician—receive midwifery care.

In the Netherlands, a country with one of the world's lowest infant-mortality rates, midwives care for nearly all pregnant and laboring women. In fact, the Dutch government, which pays for medical services for about 70 percent of the population, will not pay for a physician unless they are convinced that the mother has a medical complication needing a physician's attention.

Other countries with low infant-mortality rates, including Finland, Denmark, Norway, and Switzerland, also have a high proportion of midwife-attended births.

Of course, other factors, such as good nutrition, may be partly responsible for the fact that these countries have such low mortality rates. However, we should not underestimate the role midwifery plays in the care of the healthy mother and child.

Midwifery care for essentially healthy mothers giving birth at home or in childbearing centers is as safe, if not safer, than obstetric care in the hospital. Some physicians claim that midwifery care, particularly at home birth, is fraught with a higher percentage of medical problems and deaths than physician care in the hospital. However, studies show the very opposite! People who claim physician-attended hospital birth is safer usually base their assumption on unskilled midwifery care (which isn't really midwifery care at all) and unsupervised birth at home. As medical statistician David Stewart, PhD, points out: "Raw data for 'out-of-hospital births' are always worse than for hospitals. This is because such data usually include accidents on the way to the hospital, miscarriages at home, economically mandated home births, and even homicide (pregnant teenagers giving birth unattended and leaving their babies to die of exposure)."

To illustrate the comparative safety of midwifery care, a study of 3,257 out-of-hospital births attended by Arizona licensed midwives from 1978 to 1985 showed a perinatal mortality of 2.2 per thousand and a neonatal mortality rate of 1.1 per thousand. (The perinatal mortality rate refers to the combined total of fetal deaths occurring on or after 28 weeks of gestation.) By comparison, the U.S. infant mortality rate for 1987 was 10.5 per thousand. Similarly, a study of midwifery care in Holmes County, Mississippi showed that the infant mortality rates were almost cut in half (from thirty-eight to twenty per thousand) two years after certified nurse-midwives began providing primary care to pregnant women.

The certified nurse-midwives of the Maternity Center in Bethesda, Maryland have been attending the births of twenty to twenty-five carefully selected mothers monthly. They attended exclusively home births from 1975 to 1982 and then began attending childbearing-center births as well. Today, about three-quarters of the births take place in the center and about twenty-five percent at home. "Among all of the out-of-hospital births," says Mary Hammond-Tooke, CNM of the Maternity Center, "there have been no maternal deaths and we have never had a baby die as a result of the planned place of birth." The only perinatal deaths resulted from unavoidable problems such as severe congenital abnormalities that would have occurred in the hospital as well.

One of the most fascinating communities supporting natural childbirth and midwifery is The Farm in Summertown, Tennessee. The Farm is a spiritual and agricultural community where all births are attended by midwives who call themselves empirical midwives. Though all the midwives are experienced and skilled, none have medical training. The midwives' statistics probably remain unmatched by any hospital in the world. Of one thousand mothers who gave birth at The Farm between 1970 and 1979, the perinatal mortality rate was fifteen per thousand (this includes mothers who were transferred to the hospital). By comparison, the rate for Tennessee during this time period was twenty per thousand. Only 4 percent of the mothers were transferred to the hospital, and the cesarean-section rate was 1.5 percent.

Experienced, skilled midwives have health statistics superior to the national average even when working with high-risk clients in both home and hospital settings. Midwives usually take care of low-risk clients, referring those at high risk of pregnancy or labor complications to obstetricians. In light of this, it isn't surprising that midwives might have better health statistics.

However, numerous medical studies have shown that midwifery care has also had a dramatic impact on improving the health of high-risk mothers and babies. In a wide variety of settings, midwives are associated with a reduced incidence of low birth weight, prematurity, and neonatal mortality.

The population of North Central Bronx Hospital is comprised of a large percentage of black and Hispanic mothers, many of whom are at high risk of complications. Medical intervention is at a minimum; for example, membranes are not artificially ruptured, pain-relief medication and regional anesthesia are administered in less than 30 percent of births, and Pitocin is used to augment labor in only 3 percent of cases. Eighty-five percent of mothers give birth in a semisitting position without stirrups, and forceps are used in less than 3 percent of births. The prevailing philosophy of the midwives at this hospital includes providing emotional support through labor as well as affording the mother the freedom to eat, drink, and walk around during labor.

What are the results of this sort of midwifery care? According to medical statistician Dr. David Stewart, "With a population of mothers at considerably higher than average risk, the midwives of North Central Bronx have achieved better maternal and infant out-comes than the rest of New York City, the State of New York in gen-eral, and the United States as a whole. There isn't a single hospital in the entire country with populations of similar risk run by doctors with results as good as this one run by midwives."

A revealing study done in Madera County, California also makes a dramatic case for midwifery. In this study, the health statis-tics of obstetricians, family physicians, and nurse-midwives are compared. The results are eye-opening, to say the least. The mothers at Madera County Hospital are comprised of a high percentage of poor agricultural workers at high risk for complications. In 1959, when the hospital was staffed by family physicians, the neonatal mortality rate was a high 23.9 per thousand births. (The neonatal mortality rate refers to deaths occurring during the first twenty-eight days of life per thousand births.) From 1960 to 1963, nurse-midwives were brought in by the State of California and the neona-tal mortality rate plummeted to less than one-third, to 10.3 per thousand. Despite the fact that the population was high-risk, this statistic was better than the average for the entire state!

When obstetricians began to replace the midwives in 1964, the neonatal mortality rate more than tripled, to 32.1 per thousand! The results of this study are so astounding that one might think of it as an isolated case. However, both certified nurse-midwives and direct-entry midwives have had similar striking health statistics throughout the world.

The well-known Frontier Nursing Service (FNS) is a legend among examples of the impressively good health statistics of mid-wifery care among a high-risk clientele. FNS was founded in 1925 by Mary Breckenridge, who brought British-trained nurse-midwives to Kentucky to provide maternity care for people living in a rural area. Their statistics were tabulated by the Metropolitan Life Insur-ance Company. Between 1925 and 1951, Frontier Nursing Service midwives provided maternity care for 8,596 women. Of these,

6,533 gave birth at home, primarily in somewhat primitive conditions; the maternal death rate was only 1.2 per thousand. Though that is high by today's standards, it was one-third the maternal mortality rate for the United States as a whole at that time, which was 3.4 per thousand. The neonatal mortality rate for the early 1950s was less than the average for Kentucky and the United States as a whole.

In 1985, the Institute of Medicine published a comprehensive report about ways to prevent low birth weight, a major cause of neonatal morbidity. The report says that certified nurse-midwives were found to be particularly effective managing the care of women who are high-risk because of social and economic factors. The Institute of Medicine suggests that the superior results midwives achieve with high-risk clients may be because midwives relate to their patients in a nonauthoritarian manner, and emphasize education, emotional support, and client satisfaction. As a result, women are more likely to keep prenatal-care appointments with nurse-midwives than with physicians. The Institute of Medicine also proposed that midwives' hospital privileges be increased.

Why Are Midwifery Statistics So Impressive?

Why do skilled, experienced midwives have such outstanding health statistics? How can midwives often boast of better health statistics than obstetricians? There is no single answer. However, in addition to the reasons already given, there are a number of others.

Most midwives do not routinely use medical intervention, such as electronic fetal monitoring. Interventive obstetrics is reserved for those who need it. Researcher Dr. Lewis Mehl compared a matched population of 2,092 home- and hospital-birth mothers in the states of Wisconsin and California. Lay midwives attended 31 percent of the home births, nurse-midwives attended 2 percent, and family physicians attended 67 percent. Among hospital births, obstetricians attended 75 percent and family physicians attended 25 percent. In the hospital group, the fetal distress rate was *six* times higher than among the home-birth group. There was also triple the incidence of maternal hemorrhage, more than triple the number of babies in need of resuscitation, and quadruple the number of neonatal infections, and there were thirty permanent birth injuries caused by physicians (primarily resulting from the use of forceps).

Many midwives understand the emotional as well as the physical needs of the laboring woman. As a result, the midwife often has something I call an "opening presence"—that is, the midwife's personality and the nurturing care he or she provides encourages the mother to surrender to labor, thereby facilitating its progress.

Most midwives remain with the mother throughout labor. Studies have shown that continuous emotional support can reduce the pain, the length, and the incidence of complications in labor.

PHYSICIAN BACKUP AND HOSPITAL PRIVILEGES

All midwives should have a collaborative relationship with physicians for consultation and referral. This is essential for maternal–infant health. A physician should be readily available should complications require a doctor's care. However, many midwives, particularly direct-entry midwives, cannot find a physician willing to back them up. In the words of one physician who supports midwifery care: "The focus should be on the patient, not the practitioner. When we deny backup to midwives, we are telling the patient she doesn't have the right to the medical care she chooses. And we are denying her the health care to which every person is entitled."

Professor Helen Varney Burst, of the Maternal-Newborn Program at Yale University, says that CNMs need to be able to admit clients to the hospital, practice the full scope of midwifery within the hospital, and discharge clients. CNMs who practice in childbearing centers or homes also need full hospital privileges so that they can accompany women needing to be transferred and provide continuity of care.

I believe the midwife–physician relationship should be a mutual one entered into by equals, not one in which the physician has supervisory powers. Ideally, the midwife should function autonomously, creating her own rules and protocol. Allowing physicians to control the practice and privileges of midwives seems to me like organized restraint of trade.

LEGAL ISSUES, LICENSING, AND ACCREDITATION

Certified nurse-midwives are licensed to practice in all fifty states of the United States. However, in some states, CNMs are given privileges in only a handful of hospitals. In other states, such as California, New York, and Florida, large numbers of certified nurse-midwives work in hospitals. Every year more hospitals open their doors to midwives.

Direct-entry midwives are governed by regulations that vary dramatically from state to state within the United States. In a few states, lay midwives can be licensed, registered, or certified; however, the practices they can perform vary with the state. For example, in New Hampshire, lay midwives can be certified to offer prenatal care, assistance during labor, and postpartum care. Their practice is regulated by the New Hampshire Department of Health and Human Services. In order to become certified, they must meet state requirements for training and for clinical and home birth experience as well as pass an exam. Once certified, they may practice in both home and free-standing birth centers. Meanwhile, lay midwives who are not certified can also practice legally.

In some states, there are no laws governing direct-entry midwives; the midwives of these states are self-regulating. For example, in Vermont, where direct-entry midwives call themselves "independent midwives," midwifery is neither legal nor illegal. There is no state certification or licensing board. However, midwife Laurie Foster, who practices in both Vermont and New Hampshire, points out, "The Vermont Midwives Alliance has its own standards of protocol which are quite similar to the standards for the state of New Hampshire."

In Arizona, direct-entry midwives are also called "licensed midwives." They are licensed by the Department of Health Services, after having completed an approved course of instruction and passed state-administered exams, to provide care for essentially normal women and their newborns consisting of prenatal care, assisting in home and childbearing-center birth, and providing postpartum care and follow-up in the home after birth.

In most states, direct-entry midwives attend only home births, though they can also provide care in childbearing centers in a few locations. In 1990, U.S. direct-entry midwives began applying for hospital privileges.

In states where the practice of lay midwifery is illegal, midwives who provide much-needed obstetrical care do so at risk of fines and even imprisonment.

Changing Laws

Laws regulating midwifery practice are changing rapidly throughout the United States. Some of these laws desperately need change.

For example, not long ago in Massachusetts, a state infamous for peculiar laws, it was illegal for a certified nurse-midwife to attend a home birth but legal for another professional, say, for example, a plumber, to do so. The law has since been changed. In other states, midwives who have better health statistics than physicians have been fined and even imprisoned for practicing.

Laws making the practice of lay midwifery legal can work to the good and to the bad for the midwife and his or her clients. Legislation protects the consumer by establishing minimal standards of competency. However, it can also tie the midwife's hands by prohibiting the use of drugs, requiring collaboration and backup by physicians, and so on.

As of 1990, the ACNM is the only nationally recognized certifying organization for midwives in the United States. All nationally certified midwives are certified nurse-midwives. However, midwives are actively working toward getting official recognition for direct-entry midwives.

OPPOSITION TO MIDWIVES

Some physicians respect the services midwives are providing, while others disagree with the very idea of midwifery. Certified nurse-midwife Elizabeth Clifton, who runs a birthing center in Missouri, says, "The medical profession considers midwives of any stripe—whether they be lay midwives, certified nurse midwives, or have a PhD behind their name—absolute anathema."

Though this statement is hardly true nationwide, it does reflect the feelings of physicians in some areas. There are still thousands of hospitals across the country where CNMs cannot practice. In the words of Ernest L. Boyer, President of the Carnegie Foundation for the Advancement of Teaching, "Midwives have been subjected to a relentless campaign of innuendo and invective, a maliciously destructive crusade that not only challenged their professional competence, but debased their character as well."

The opposition to midwifery—ranging from prejudice based on ignorance to outright persecution—reminds me of the response physicians made to Ignaz Phillip Semmelweiss, the first physician to demonstrate statistically the cause of puerperal fever. When Dr. Semmelweiss, a Viennese physician, observed that the mortality rate of mothers in the medical students' ward was 437 percent greater than the rate in the midwives' ward, he concluded that doctors were transmitting the disease. He also discovered the cure: antiseptic hand-washing. Doctors ridiculed him for this, refusing to believe what the statistics clearly showed. One respected physician even argued that physicians were gentlemen whose hands were clean.

The epidemic of puerperal fever is a thing of the past, but the attitude of physicians is not. Many doctors still refuse to pay attention to the statistics that show midwifery care is as safe as—if not safer than—physicians care. Like the doctors in nineteenth-century Vienna, they are still ridiculing those who show us how to reduce infant and maternal disease.

Why the Opposition?

Given midwifery's superior health statistics, one would think all health professionals would unanimously welcome midwives, that they would increase government support of midwifery care, and that hospitals would improve their backup services for home-birth midwives. Yet the very opposite is the case, despite the fact that support of midwifery is obviously in the best interests of maternal and child health.

In some cases, the prejudice against midwives is based on ignorance. Many physicians fear midwives lack both education and high standards of practice. While it is true that many direct-entry midwives are not regulated by a certification board or committee of healthcare professionals, and a few lack skills and experience, most midwives offer very high standards of maternity care. Other physicians hold the genuine belief that obstetricians provide safer care for mothers and babies. Despite information to the contrary published in their own journals, many obstetricians (and parents) are so firmly entrenched in the belief that mothers need technological intervention to birth safely that facts don't seem to persuade them otherwise.

Another reason for the prejudice may be that midwives and physicians are essentially competing for the same middle- to upper-class clients. As one physician puts it: "Those physicians who see CNMs as a threat to the pocketbook take refuge behind all kinds of philosophical and medical baloney." Midwives can offer equal if not superior health care at less cost than obstetricians. The motive behind some physicians' opposition may simply be to eliminate competition. Dr. David Stewart, founder of The International Association for Parents and Professionals for Safe Alternatives in Childbirth (NAPSAC), says that the "dramatic disappearance of a centuries-old profession, almost to extinction, was no accident."

Meanwhile, opposition to midwifery is not entirely one-sided. A few midwives have been equally hostile toward the medical profession. A handful of vocal midwives seem to be waging an angry campaign against what they perceive as the male-dominated medical establishment, and a small number oppose medical care of any kind. Fortunately for mothers, these midwives represent a tiny minority.

Nothing can be accomplished with hostility. The goal of safe alternative births in the setting and manner in which mothers choose can be widely achieved only if all childbirth professionals—midwives, physicians, childbirth educators, and nurses, male and female—accept, respect, and support one another's work.

A FINAL NOTE

The increasing popularity of the midwife—including physicians and naturopaths who practice like midwives—is perhaps the single greatest stride forward for alternative birth.

If current trends in midwifery continue, certified nurse-midwives will grow in number and become even more popular than they are today. The outdated hospitals that now deny nurse-midwives privileges will either open the doors to this increasingly popular childbirth professional or succumb to their competitors. I believe we will also soon welcome a new professional to the established system of medical care. Direct-entry midwives will not only grow in numbers; they will become legitimate, their practice recognized, and their work respected throughout the United States.

Perhaps midwifery will become the standard of maternity care throughout the nation. If this happens, we will no doubt see a dramatic change. As direct-entry midwife Joan Remington asserts, "Midwives will make their mark! There is no doubt we will have a significant impact on lowering perinatal mortality as every study, the experiences of every midwifery practice in the U.S. and overseas, has proven over and over."

In addition, there will be a greater focus on the emotional

needs of the family throughout the childbearing drama. This, in turn, will spell more positive birth experiences for the entire family. The midwife will once again become what he or she has always been since the dawn of history: an integral figure in maternal–child health care throughout the world.

And you and your baby will benefit.

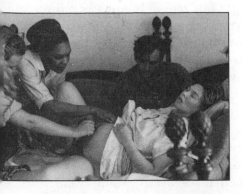

CHAPTER 5

Birth at Home

OUR FIRST SON, CARL, WAS BORN
in a hospital, where my wife, Jan, had first-rate medical care. The
obstetrician who attended the birth, Leo Sorger, M.D., is one of the
most prominent and highly skilled in New England. He is also one
of those rare physicians who is fully committed to helping parents
give birth the way they choose. The dimly lit room where Carl was
born was peaceful, pleasant, and comfortable. The birth was one of
the peak experiences of our lives. Yet we decided to give birth to our
next child at home.

Despite our positive in-hospital experience, we couldn't dis-
miss the fact that leaving our comfortable home in the middle of the
night to go to a hospital, a place associated with sickness, had been
unnecessarily traumatic. Beginning a family is a tremendously emotional time for the new parents—to say nothing of the baby. We felt
it should take place at home.

When our second son was born, we were living in an apartment in Brookline, Massachusetts. Since our apartment never quite
felt like home, we made arrangements to rent a house on a hill in
central Vermont for his birth. There, I "caught" our son Paul, as Dr.
Thurmond Knight, a now-retired family physician, played Renaissance flute while waiting to assist if necessary.

Jan seemed far more at peace in our rented home than she had
in the hospital. "I felt more comfortable and more secure," she said.
"Also it was wonderful to be able to stay in one place throughout
labor."

Just a few miles from our rented home where Paul was born
was a hospital that had one of the most flexible birthing units I had

ever visited. Nevertheless, we chose to give birth in the mountain-top home. Dr. Louis DiNicola, a pediatrician who cares about mothers having joyful birth experiences as well as healthy babies, was incredulous: When I told him I thought our rented home was more comfortable than the hospital, he exploded: "You can't tell me that your rented house high on the top of that hill—where you are surrounded by two feet of snow and ice, where it's twenty below zero and the wind howls, where you have no central heating and you have to get up during labor to stoke up the stove with more wood—you can't tell me *that* is more comfortable than our birthing rooms! Here you have all the conveniences of home. You don't have to be concerned about changing the sheets and cleaning up. Everything you need is provided for you including absolute privacy. And you don't have to worry about medical help if you need it. I simply can't believe that the place you and your wife chose to give birth is more comfortable in any way!"

He had a point. If Jan had given birth in the birthing room, she could have had the same noninterventive care and the same peace and quiet, I could have caught the baby, and the physician could even have played the flute. And there was even a view of ancient sugar maples outside the window.

Yet there was a difference. Our rented home was *our* place—at least for the duration of our stay. And it had a personal ambience, a sense of peace, comfort, and security, that no hospital could reproduce. Not even a hospital with a view of sugar maples.

When it was time for the birth of our third son, Jonathan, we decided that, since our Brookline apartment was our real home (like it or not), we would have the baby there. Jan was attended by Sloane Crawford, CNM, a Brookline midwife who helps parents create the birth of their choice.

Few hospitals are as noisy as our bedroom was that Sunday morning between four and five A.M. Our apartment was on the second floor. During Jan's labor, our downstairs neighbor, upset about being woken, began shrieking, hollering, swearing, and pounding on the walls and finally called the police to complain about the noise! (It may have been in retaliation for my having many times phoned the police about his loud stereo.) So in addition to the noise, we had unexpected company. I remember the face of one of the policemen who came to our apartment. He arrived just after the baby was born, and though he didn't witness the birth, his face all but radiated with that near-magical glow often seen on those who witness their first birth. As he was leaving he said to his partner, "A baby! It was just born!"

Despite the noise, the interruptions, and the visitors, comparing the two home births with our hospital experience, Jan recalls: "It was more peaceful, more relaxing, better to have the family together, and better in every way to be at home."

Thousands of parents agree. Parents who have had both hospital and home births invariably describe birth at home as a more positive experience. As one mother put it: "There is simply no comparison. Hospital and home birth don't even belong in the same category!"

Birth at home was so important to one expectant mother that she was willing to travel out of state to achieve her goal. She couldn't find a physician or midwife to attend her home birth near the town where she lived in Florida, so she temporarily relocated to her grandmother's house in Alabama, where a midwife was willing to assist her. She describes her experience: "I was able to give birth in the same bed where my grandmother gave birth to all her five children, including my mother. Everyone in the room was crying tears of joy, but the tears that touched me the most were those of my big, strong husband as he held me and his baby boy. . . . We just couldn't go to sleep. We lay there for thirty minutes talking about the birth and about how happy we were. We couldn't wipe the smiles off our faces. It was so sweet and gentle and special. That is one thing I wish I had a picture of, although the picture will never leave my mind."

THE SAFETY OF HOME BIRTH

Prior to the turn of the century, 95 percent of Americans were born at home. By 1940, half of the population were still giving birth outside of hospital settings. In 1990, only 2 to 3 percent of U.S. mothers gave birth in their own home. However, for an increasing number home is becoming the birth place of choice.

Ann and Dennis, who chose home birth for both their children, echo the feelings of other home-birth parents: "After much research we felt we would actually be safer at home."

As Phillip G. Stubblefield, M.D., Associate Professor of Obstetrics and Gynecology of Harvard Medical School, puts it: "If the mother can be transported to a hospital within ten minutes where a team awaits capable of performing an emergency cesarean section, the outcome of an emergency at home may be better than if the mother were laboring in a small hospital where it would take half a hour to assemble the cesarean-section team. In addition, there is evidence that at the extreme, the cold, overly professional atmosphere of the worst hospital settings may increase obstetric casualties."

Unfortunately, research on the safety of home birth is limited. However, the few published medical and statistical studies have shown that for *selected, healthy mothers*, home birth is associated with lower cesarean rates, fewer complications, and optimum family–infant bonding.

In 1976 Dr. Lewis Mehl and his associates compared 1,046 home births with the same number of hospital births. Both groups were matched for maternal age, length of pregnancy, number of past births, risk factors, education, and socioeconomic status. There was no difference in infant mortality between the two groups. However, among the hospital births there was significantly more cases of intrauterine fetal distress, elevated blood pressure during labor, lacerations, postpartum hemorrhage, birth injuries, neonatal infection, and babies in need of resuscitation. In the hospital, obstetric pain-relief medication was used more frequently. Many more forceps deliveries were done, more cesareans were performed, and nine times as many episiotomies were cut. These complications may have been *iatrogenic*, that is, physician-caused. They may have resulted from obstetric intervention or perhaps from the hospital environment.

In another study, Dr. Mehl and his associates compared planned home births attended by midwives with physician-attended planned hospital births. The mothers were matched for age, education, number of pregnancies, length of gestation, presentation (the baby's position in relation to the mother's pelvis), and risk status. The researchers found no significant differences in perinatal mortality, birth weight, or other major complications. However, when compared to the hospital births, the home births were associated with higher Apgar scores (a test of the baby's color, pulse, respiration, muscle tone, and reflexes), less fetal distress, fewer incidents of postpartum hemorrhage, fewer birth injuries, and less need for infant resuscitation.

Working with psychotherapist Gayle Peterson and P.H. Leiderman, Dr. Mehl also found that undrugged home birth may have an improved psychological maternal outcome over anesthetized hospital birth. They state: "Anesthetized hospital delivery was found to have a humiliating effect with decreases in self-worth and self-esteem whereas natural hospital, and more so, home delivery, tended to increase self-worth and self-esteem. More symptoms of postpartum depression were present in anesthetized hospital deliveries and decreased in the continuum from an anesthetized hospital to home delivery."

An extensive analysis of over 3,200 births attended by Arizona's licensed midwives over the past eight years also shows impressive results. The perinatal mortality rate was 2.2 per thousand, which includes three deaths resulting from congenital abnormalities. Researchers Deborah A. Sullivan and Rose Weitz, associate professors of sociology at Arizona State University, state that this analysis, though not conclusive, "does suggest that there is little, if any, risk involved in choosing midwife-attended out-of-hospital birth in Arizona."

However, many parents and professionals still believe that hospital birth is associated with increased safety for mother and child. There *was* a dramatic reduction in maternal and fetal mortality when the place of birth shifted from home to hospital in this country, but this does not mean the hospital was responsible for the improvement. Other factors such as better prenatal care, better nutrition, fewer low-birth-weight babies, the availability of antibiotics, and better diagnosis of complications were also involved.

There is no evidence to suggest that home birth is associated with any more risk of neonatal death than hospital birth. Indeed, as has been seen, studies show a lower incidence. Bear in mind, however, that this does not necessarily mean home birth has less medical risk than hospital birth. The better statistics in home-birth studies also result from the fact that a lower-risk population plans home births in the first place.

Both professionals and the general public have been swayed by misleading information about home birth. For example, in 1978 the American College of Obstetricians and Gynecologists (ACOG) issued a news release that claimed, on the basis of information gathered from eleven state health departments, that the risk to the baby's life was two to five times greater in out-of-hospital birth than in hospital birth. Another study published in the *American Journal of Obstetrics and Gynecology* gives similar statistics.

However, neither of these studies distinguishes between planned and unplanned out-of-hospital births. Unplanned out-of-hospital births include late miscarriages, premature births, precipitous (that is, sudden, unplanned) deliveries, and unattended home births. The majority of the unplanned births were precipitous deliveries. This complication is associated with about a seven-times greater incidence of low birth weight, which in turn is associated with increased perinatal mortality. A world of difference separates the planned home births from the emergency delivery in the car!

Meanwhile, bear in mind that a carefully planned home birth includes a sensible choice of caregiver. Home-birth advocates including Dr. Mehl and his associates are quick to point out that there are many stories of women who have witnessed one or two births, then call themselves midwives. Remember, there is a great difference between experienced, trained midwives and people only calling themselves midwives.

Does home birth present any risk? Unexpected life-threatening complications *do* occur during home birth. There is always an element of risk. As pediatrician Dr. Louis DiNicola puts it: "Home birth carries a risk for both mother and baby. Acute emergencies like maternal hemorrhaging or fetal asphyxia can arise during labor and delivery without warning. Such require immediate medical attention which is not always possible at home."

The major complications that are better handled in a hospital than at home include placental abruption, umbilical-cord prolapse, maternal postpartum hemorrhage, and neonatal asphyxia. The home-birth practitioner's screening process and methods of managing labor reduce the likelihood and severity of some of these. If, in spite of the best care, one of these complications develops, a competent midwife or physician is usually able to manage the problem.

Alice Bailes, CNM, a midwife in Alexandria, Virginia who has attended 700 home births, says she has rarely encountered a baby with difficulty breathing requiring her to use her emergency oxygen for a few seconds to help the baby along. However, she points out: "We don't deliver premature babies, babies of smokers, and mothers with high blood pressure; we don't give drugs that might compromise the baby's ability to breathe. We listen to the baby's heart tones often and carefully through labor. If we hear variations that do not respond well to maternal position changes, we consider transferring the mother to a hospital where a neonatal team is ready in case of respiratory distress."

For healthy mothers, the risk is small. But as home-birth practitioners Drs. Sagov and Feinbloom point out: "Families must be informed of this very small but real risk, which they must balance against the risks, largely iatrogenic and psychological, incurred in the hospital."

No one can tell a mother she is perfectly safe giving birth at home. Whether she is safer at home than in a hospital, however, is another question. I'll always remember how one obstetrician (who practices in both a hospital and homes) answered my own question when Jan and I were considering whether or not to give birth at home: "If you ask me if home birth is a risk, I have to say yes. If you ask me what I would do if it were my child, despite the risk, my answer would be: Give birth at home."

Which is what we did.

THE ADVANTAGES OF HOME BIRTH

Parents elect to give birth at home for a wide variety of reasons.

For Kathy Kangas, who later founded Childbirth Education Services in Worcester County, Massachusetts, it was dissatisfaction with the hospital where she had given birth to her first child, Amanda: "Even though we carefully chose our obstetrician and discussed what I wanted—no IV, no monitor, no episiotomy, and so on—when we got to the hospital, it was a major war to get what I wanted. So when my husband, Tyler, and I got pregnant the next time, our first inclination was to give birth at home. I began to study about childbirth. It wasn't long before I was convinced that staying home was not only more comfortable but safer, and that it was a risk to go to the hospital and get all that intervention or have to fight not to have it."

"Home birth," says Dr. DiNicola, "is a symptom of the failure of the medical profession to provide appropriate care for healthy mothers and babies. In hospitals, almost everything is done for the convenience of the physician and delivery room personnel, not for the comfort of mother and child."

While dissatisfaction with hospital birth is one of the primary reasons parents choose to give birth at home, it is by no means the only reason. Practitioners who have attended both home and hospital births have noted that birth at home may enable the mother to respond more positively to labor. For example, Vermont physician Dr. Thurmond Knight observes: "The quality of labor is often utterly different at home than in a hospital. A woman's strength comes out at a home birth and she is able to welcome the changes that take place in her body. She is in the most natural place to have a baby—the place where she feels most comfortable and secure. She is able to make her own decisions rather than submit to protocol. And she is surrounded by loved ones—guests in her home—not strangers who control an unfamiliar setting."

There are many advantages to childbirth at home.

At home the parents are in complete control. One of the central themes common to a large number of home-birth parents is the desire to reclaim control over the childbearing experience. In her own home, the mother does not have to relinquish control of her birth experience to medical staff. "One reason I had a home birth is that I wanted to be the one who led the show," recalls one mother, "not have someone else tell me what I could or couldn't do."

Many women today want to reassert control over their bodies and their medical care. California nurse-midwife June Whitson, who assists at both birth-center and home births, says, "Only at home does the mother feel in charge of what she is doing. By acknowledging that we feel comfortable helping a woman give birth at home, we birth attendants are telling her that we trust her body and her instincts to do what is best in order to have her baby in the safest, most comfortable way."

At home, the mother does not have to assert herself to get the kind of medical care she wants. During labor a woman is highly sensitive and vulnerable. This is no time to have to stand up for your rights and fight for the kind of birth you want. "It's your baby, your body," affirms childbirth educator Mariann Martinez of Mystic, Connecticut. "You shouldn't have to fight for what is already yours."

The mother is free to do whatever she wants during labor. She is free to eat, drink, get up and walk around, and give birth in the position of her choice. She does not have to confront impersonal hospital policies, such as the policy of withholding light meals and liquids from laboring women. She is able to devote all her attention to her labor, not to adapting to someone else's schedule or routines.

Certified nurse-midwife Alice Bailes attended a birth where the mother moaned, groaned, and grunted quite loudly during labor. Between her contractions, the mother broke into a big smile and said, "I'm glad I'm home where I can feel comfortable about making these loud sounds without worrying about offending or disturbing anyone." Her six-year-old and two-and-a-half-year-old children started grunting along with her when she pushed the baby out into the world.

The mother can invite whomever she wants to be with her. This is a basic human right not protected by law. Many hospitals restrict the number of people the mother can have with her during labor.

The caregivers are guests in the mother's home. Lisa Jensen, licensed New Hampshire midwife, considers this one of the major differences between home and hospital birth. "The home birth practitioner is a visitor present at the parents' invitation," she says, "not an authority who is in charge." Many parents appreciate this difference.

Howard Marchbanks, M.D., a Southern California physician who attends home, childbearing-center, and hospital births, tells his clients, "I always feel I am a special guest in your home, whom you have invited to attend the special occasion of your birth."

The mother does not have to have unfamiliar or unsupportive persons present. "What if the nurse is unsupportive or you simply don't get along?" says one new mother who chose to give birth at home. "Sure, you can ask for a change if there is another nurse available. But doing that can open the door for you to be treated coldly throughout the rest of labor."

The mother is able to avoid unnecessary medical intervention, such as the routine use of intravenous feeding (IV), electronic fetal monitoring (EFM), and hormonal augmentation of labor if she doesn't give birth within an allotted time frame. As I discussed in Chapter One, the injudicious use of medical intervention may cause complications and increase the chance of having a cesarean section.

The risk of infection is reduced for both mother and baby. During pregnancy, the baby receives antibodies from the mother via the placenta. These antibodies provide immunities to familiar family germs, making home-born babies less likely to contract bacterial or viral diseases such as urinary-tract infection. Hospitals are public places that house collections of unfamiliar and sometimes virulent pathogens that can cause infections in both mother and baby.

Many mothers feel more comfortable laboring at home than in a clinical environment. At home the mother is on her own familiar turf—the ideal place to begin her family. As Mariann Martinez, childbirth educator and mother, puts it: "I never considered going to a hospital to have a baby. I don't feel that birth is an illness. The hospital is a place for people who have problems."

The mother does not have to move from one place to another during labor. While being up and about can facilitate labor's progress, moving from one's home to the hospital may have just the opposite effect and cause labor to slow down. It's rather an odd custom—liking moving from one place to another during lovemaking, it can be done, but it's seldom the most comfortable or effective way.

Parents and baby are not separated. After a home birth, the immediate postpartum period is usually less traumatic for the baby as well as the mother. Parents and infant can enjoy immediate and prolonged bonding time without interruption. Breastfeeding and parent–infant contact are not interrupted by having the baby weighed, measured, or examined. These procedures can be postponed as long as the parents want and then done in the presence of family.

Home is the only place some parents can have the birth experience they really want. If you would like to have siblings at birth, have the father "catch" the baby, or have a midwife-attended delivery, you may not be able to find a childbearing center or hospital to accommodate your plans.

Home birth is a fraction of the cost of birth in the hospital. The parents avoid the hospital fee, a significant portion of maternity-care cost. This is especially attractive to parents who don't have optimum health-care insurance.

Yet another advantage of home birth is the special, almost magical beauty a hospital can't create no matter how comfortable the environment or how positive the staff. In the words of Dr. Knight: "Births I've witnessed in parents' homes are the most beautiful and holy I've ever attended. Nothing equals home for peace and privacy. Home is unquestionably the best place for normal labor and birth, providing a woman is healthy."

Interestingly, Dr. Knight was trained in a conventional Florida hospital where, like most American physicians, he had never witnessed an alternative birth. A neighbor invited him to attend her home birth in the role of a friend, not a practitioner, and that birth was the turning point of his career. The home birth was unlike anything he had ever witnessed in a hospital. "The way I had looked at deliveries in the past had no meaning after this home birth," he recalls. "In the holy silence of that farmhouse bedroom, I had seen what childbirth was meant to be."

THE DISADVANTAGES OF HOME BIRTH

Despite the many benefits of childbirth at home, there are a few disadvantages to weigh and consider.

- *Home birth is limited to the low-risk mother.* The mother with medical complications cannot safely give birth at home.
- *Home-birth services are not available everywhere.* In some areas, the parents are not able to find a competent home-birth practitioner.
- *Home birth is not widely accepted by the medical establishment.* The parents who choose this childbirth alternative risk the disapproval of some health professionals and even of relatives and friends.
- *It is not possible, even with careful screening, to guarantee that any particular mother is low-risk.* Problems can always develop at the last minute that are impossible to predict in advance.
- *There is no effective way to provide rapid emergency delivery in the home environment.* For example, if a problem such as severe fetal distress arises, requiring an emergency cesarean, the mother must be transported to the hospital immediately. This cannot be assured unless the out-of-hospital birth environment is located very close by.
- *Blood transfusions cannot be effectively done in the out-of-hospital setting.*

FACTORS INCREASING THE RISK OF BIRTH AT HOME

The mother with any of the following is probably safest giving birth in a hospital.

- diabetes (depending on the severity of the condition)
- high blood pressure
- heart disease
- kidney disease
- an *active* case of genital herpes at the time of labor
- anemia that persists until the time of delivery
- Rh-negative blood with antibody sensitization (a blood incompatibility presenting a risk to the baby)
- unexplained bleeding during pregnancy
- preeclampsia
- polyhydramnios or oligohydramnios (too much or too little amniotic fluid)
- premature labor
- postmature labor
- multiple pregnancy
- baby in the breech position
- history of previous unexplained stillbirth
- history of hemorrhage (many caregivers will assess the reason for hemorrhage, as this condition is frequently iatrogenic)
- any other condition for which hospitalization may be advisable

Bear in mind that there are risks in a hospital birth as well. For most home-birth parents, the disadvantages of home birth are outweighed by the benefits.

IS HOME BIRTH FOR YOU?

Parents from a wide variety of backgrounds—from farmers to physicians—elect to give birth at home.

The first thing to ask yourself is whether you feel comfortable about giving birth at home. Whether you opt for home, childbearing center, or hospital, you are most likely to labor efficiently if you are comfortable in your birthing environment. Learning as much as you can about each will help you determine which setting seems most congenial.

The next thing to determine is whether or not home birth is safe for you. Practitioners vary in their criteria for determining who can give birth at home with relative safety, but most agree with the following qualifications:

- The mother should be in good health.
- She should be attended by a well-trained physician or midwife with adequate medical supplies, including oxygen and resuscitation equipment.
- She should be prepared to leave her home and go to the nearest medical facility should complications develop.
- Her home should be located within a ten- to fifteen-minute drive of a hospital. The mother who lives farther from the hospital may want to consider a childbearing center. Lacking a nearby childbirth center, a few parents have temporarily relocated to a friend's home or even a hotel suite near a medical facility.

All practitioners also agree that the home-birth candidate should be carefully screened to be sure she is *low-risk*. The mother with pregnancy complications such as high blood pressure or who has any of the other risk factors listed on page 118 is probably better off giving birth in the hospital with the latest medical equipment readily available. Low and high risk, however, are relative terms. Some health professionals are overly stringent in their definition of low risk, as has been seen. If you don't agree with your caregiver's opinion about your risk status, get a second opinion.

It's important to take responsibility for planning your birth carefully and for becoming as well-informed and as well-educated about childbirth as possible. You'll probably need to work a little harder should you elect home birth, because it is not yet widely accepted in this country. Preparation is often more difficult than preparation for hospital birth. Depending on where your home is located, you may have to search longer for a competent caregiver. You will have to purchase many of your own supplies and locate a backup hospital should a transfer be necessary. This chapter will help you accomplish that.

Several studies have been done to describe the type of parents who choose home birth. For the most part, home-birth parents do not differ in educational or socioeconomic background from other mothers, although several studies have found that women choosing home birth are more highly educated than others. Most consider their options carefully before making a choice. As Elizabeth Hosford, CNM, past coordinator of the Maternity Center Association in New York City, observes: "In many ways home-birth couples are in the forefront with other who are leading the way toward greater individual responsibility for health. They are keenly interested and highly motivated."

As a general rule, home-birth parents tend to have philosophical differences from their hospital-birth counterparts. Most view childbirth as a normal, healthy process, emphasize the importance of family bonding and participation, and believe that parents should take personal responsibility for their own and their children's health care. Most home-birth parents also breastfeed, another vital health advantage to the newborn.

Planning a home birth includes

- making a decision
- choosing a home-birth caregiver
- providing for an emergency backup physician (if your caregiver hasn't already arranged this)
- choosing a backup hospital
- getting home-birth supplies

MAKING THE DECISION

Like many couples, Cheri and Martin didn't begin to investigate their options until Cheri was six months pregnant. She was dissatisfied with her obstetrician, who gave offhand responses to many of her questions. A friend had spoken highly of her own home birth. "We were both unsure about it," recalls Cheri. "I began to read everything I could in the library about childbirth." After she and Martin weighed their options, she was convinced that it was better to have the baby at home.

Another couple, Jean and Tony, who have two sons and two daughters, didn't learn about home birth until after their first daughter was born in a hospital. Jean says: "I didn't have my first child at home because at the time I didn't even realize you could do that! My

husband was a little unsure about home birth at first. But after reading and praying about it we felt home birth was right for us."

Ideally, you and your mate should jointly make the decision to
give birth at home. If both parents are in agreement, anxiety and
negative feelings in the birth place will be reduced.

Make your choice with care. "Having the baby at home now
seems normal and natural to me, but the decision to do so was not
made easily," says Bill, a father of two in East Texas. His wife,
Linda, considered a home birth largely to avoid another cesarean
section. She recalls: "The more we read, the more we felt certain
our chances at being permitted to have a vaginal birth were very
slight in our local hospital, which had a cesarean section rate of 25
percent. Once the decision was made it was like a weight had been
lifted from my shoulders. I was able to feel exuberant about this
pregnancy. I was thrilled with the sense of control I regained." (Depending on the type of uterine incision, vaginal birth after a previous cesarean is usually quite safe. If you have had a cesarean,
check with your physician or midwife to be sure vaginal delivery
will be safe for you.)

As more parents are educated about home birth, more will
elect this option. Many do not choose home birth because they are
simply unaware that it is an option or don't realize what it offers.

For example, Tami Michele, a childbirth educator in Grand-
ville, Michigan, says, "I had the typical American attitude of 'I believe birth is a natural physiological body function, but it's best to
have a baby in the hospital in case anything goes wrong.'" For this
reason, she gave birth to her first two children in the hospital. Then
a couple in one of her childbirth classes decided to have a baby at
home with a midwife, and the parents asked Tami to be their labor
support person.

"I was shocked and nervous about it," Tami recalls. But she believed that it was a mother's choice to give birth in the place where
she felt most safe and supported the parents during the birth, and
her feelings were altered by the experience: "As I left their home I
had a feeling about this birth that I had never experienced before.
Each baby's birth is a miracle, but there was something so special
about this one. The midwife had a certain way of handling the birth
which I had never seen in an obstetrician or a hospital. The mother
worked with the long labor so well. And the baby had a peaceful
contentment about him, like he was glad to be here."

Tami's next two children were born at home.

HOME-BIRTH CAREGIVERS

The term *caregiver* has been used throughout this book to indicate any person who provides prenatal care, attends birth, and provides postpartum health care. Several health professionals give medical care through the childbearing season.

- *Certified nurse-midwife (CNM),* a person educated in both nursing and midwifery who is qualified to provide health care for the childbearing woman and to assist at normal births.
- *Other midwives,* persons who have been trained through various combinations of apprenticeship, midwifery school, and nursing experience.
- *Family practitioner,* a physician who practices general medicine and provides health care for the whole family.
- *Obstetrician,* a physician who specializes in delivering babies and in the diseases of childbearing women.
- *Naturopath,* a health-care provider specializing in natural healing methods. Naturopaths who attend births are not common in the United States.
- *Chiropractor,* a health-care provider who specializes in spinal adjustment. Many chiropractors are also trained in other natural healing methods, and in a few states they are licensed to attend home birth.

CHOOSING A HOME-BIRTH CAREGIVER

While guidelines for choosing a caregiver are discussed in Chapter Three, this section will give you some additional information about selecting a caregiver who specializes in home birth.

The majority of home-birth practitioners are midwives. In fact, the renaissance of midwifery in the United States is to a large part the direct result of the increasing number of parents seeking competent, supportive home-birth caregivers. Many midwives require their clients to have routine prenatal visits with a physician to screen for possible complications in addition to their own midwifery prenatal care. Most also bring an assistant with them.

Physicians do attend home births; however, they are unfortunately few and far between. In my area, the local obstetrician, who is entirely supportive of helping a mother give birth the way she wants in the hospital, will not attend a home birth. However, he recommends a lay midwife who, he admits, is more knowledgeable about home birth than he is. He will also permit the midwife to "catch" the baby if the mother must be transferred to the hospital. Or, if there are complications requiring his intervention in the hospital, the midwife may remain with the parents to give emotional support.

Dr. Howard Marchbanks of La Habra, California has the ideal approach. He attends home, childbearing-center, and hospital births. I wish all physicians would follow his example, meeting clients' needs in the birth place of their choice; this would make it a lot easier for parents to plan their birth. Dr. Marchbanks, who works with midwives, gives all his clients a brochure about nutrition, prenatal care, and other valuable information including the advantages of home, childbearing-center, and hospital birth. He is one of the only physicians I have met who gives his clients honest, objective information about all three options without attempting to influence their decision (though he does admit that he personally prefers the childbearing center because he does not have to leave his office!).

Whether midwife or physician, all competent caregivers do regular prenatal exams. This includes keeping charts on blood pressure, weight gain, blood and urine samples, and fetal growth and heartbeat. However, most home-birth practitioners spend a longer time with clients to give nutritional suggestions, ensure the normalcy of the pregnancy, and discuss concerns and emotional and psychosocial factors with the parents. The caregiver will also make at least one prenatal visit to your home to be sure you have adequate supplies, and many caregivers will also make a postpartum visit.

The caregiver who attends your birth will do a newborn exam. However, as suggested in Chapter Three, during pregnancy you should also pick out your baby's caregiver for the weeks and months following birth.

It is important to interview the caregiver. A safe home-birth practitioner will meet all of the following requirements.

Thorough training and experience. This is your primary concern. You want to be sure your practitioner can recognize complications and handle an emergency. Most midwives are well-trained and experienced, and many have better safety statistics than obstetricians. However, a few learn on the job without supervision.

Don't hesitate to ask questions. How many home births has the caregiver attended? (Some caregivers have attended less than fifty, others several hundred.) How was he or she trained? Is he or she licensed by the state or certified? What equipment does the caregiver bring? Can he or she do suturing should you need a laceration repaired? Some midwives have to call someone else to come to the home or transport mothers to the hospital should suturing be required.

Ask the practitioner how he or she handles emergency situations. You also might want to ask about his or her criteria for transferring clients to the hospital.

Adequate medical equipment. In addition to a fetoscope or doppler (a hand-held ultrasound device that amplifies the fetal heart tones), this should include oxygen for infant resuscitation, appropriate medications such as oxytocic drugs should hemorrhage occur, suturing materials, and other equipment. The practitioner may request that you purchase some supplies. For more on supplies for a home birth, see page 131.

Adequate backup by a physician. If you choose a midwife for primary caregiver, you or the midwife should have arrangements with a physician should an emergency arise requiring a physician's intervention. Access to local physician backup is a major factor in planning a safe home birth. This cannot be stressed enough.

Backup arrangements with a hospital. Should a sudden complication arise requiring a last-minute transfer, the caregiver should have arrangements to transfer you without delay.

To locate a good home-birth practitioner, talk with childbirth educators, midwives, family practitioners, and obstetricians in your area. If the caregiver you contact does not attend home births, ask for a reference. If nothing else, you will make health professionals aware that an increasing number of parents are requesting home-birth services.

Unfortunately, in areas where there are no physicians who attend home birth and there is no support for midwifery at home, you may have difficulty finding a home-birth practitioner. In such a case, consult the *NAPSAC Directory of Alternative Birth Services and Consumer Guide,* included in the Suggested Reading List at the end of this book.

GIVING BIRTH ALONE

A minority of parents give birth at home with no professional caregiver present. Those who plan in advance to give birth without a caregiver present do so for several reasons.

The parents wish to "catch" the baby themselves. Some parents choose to be unattended by a professional because they want a father-caught birth. If the parents want the father to catch the baby, they generally can plan this option with their caregiver. As I mentioned previously, I caught our second child with a physician present and our third child with a midwife present. However, some families that elect to be alone do not feel this event should be shared by a professional—particularly a person who is a relative stranger. As one mother put it: "I didn't want anyone besides my husband to touch me."

The parents are unable to create the birth of their choice any other way. They cannot find a caregiver who supports their individual plans, whether these plans involve a father-caught delivery, children at birth, or simply a home birth.

David and Lee Stewart's story is a classic example. They were unable to find a midwife or physician to attend the home births of their children, which occurred between 1962 and 1976. Their five healthy children, therefore, were all born without a professional in attendance. *(The Stewarts do not suggest that other parents follow their example.)*

Inspired by the need of parents for alternative-birth care, the Stewarts later founded the InterNational Association for Parents and Professionals for Safe Alternatives in Childbirth (NAPSAC), which now has chapters throughout the world. Today NAPSAC publishes books and pamphlets promoting safe, natural alternative-birth options. You can find their address at the end of the book.

Do-it-yourself home birth is in part the result of our society's failure to provide alternatives to those who choose them. The Association for Childbirth at Home, International (ACHI) conducted a research study on do-it-yourself home birth in southern California. Its founder and president, Tonya Brooks, says: "We found most DIY couples in southern California were educated people who have the money for and the availability of birth attendants. Their reasons for deliberately choosing a DIY were various. Many had been rudely denied care and had, thus, become radicalized against all health-care providers."

The parents feel that birth is a sacred or highly intimate experience to be shared only by a couple, or the immediate family. As one mother put it: "We simply felt that birth was and is a holy event and should be kept in the family if the pregnancy is normal and the baby is healthy."

Most home-birth advocates agree that unattended birth poses a significant risk. Parents who choose an unattended home birth have no way of monitoring fetal well-being and no way of handling emergencies should they arise. The *Journal of the American Medical Association* published a study conducted by The Center of Disease Control, Atlanta, of home births that took place in North Carolina between 1974 and 1976. Neonatal mortality rates were three per thousand for planned home births that were attended by a lay midwife, thirty per thousand for planned home births with no attendant, and 120 per thousand for unplanned home births. (By comparison, the neonatal death rate among hospital births was twelve per thousand, which included high-risk pregnancies and low-birth-weight babies. Excluding the low-birth-weight babies, the hospital neonatal death rate was seven per thousand.

The majority of parents who plan a do-it-yourself birth are aware of the risk. As one mother says: "We felt unattended home births were probably more dangerous than attended ones, but we felt that the only doctor doing them in our area wasn't competent or a man we could talk to. And I was thrown out of my previous OB's office because of my 'nonsensical ideas' about birth. After that, I read books, got a medical textbook and we decided to do it ourselves." And another mother said, "I felt the procedures I would be subjected to in the hospital were just as dangerous as an unattended home birth."

Parents who want a do-it-yourself birth are advised to have a competent health professional present to intervene only if necessary. For example, Alice Bailes, CNM, tells the story of one of her favorite "unattended" births: "When I arrived at the parents' home, the parents-to-be were working together in labor. I came into the darkened bedroom quietly, and took my place in a corner on the rug. I sat there silently for a while. Then I stood up and said, 'Excuse me, I'd like to listen to the baby.' After checking the fetal heart tones, I resumed my post in the corner. I remained there for the next hour and a half with brief sorties to the baby to hear the heart tones every twenty minutes or so.

"Then the mom moved up onto her side in the bed where her husband helped her get supported with some pillows. I took my birth set out of my bag, put my instruments in the placenta bowl, put on my gloves, and sat in a corner of the bed where I could see well. The dad sat in front of his wife while she put her knee on his shoulder.

"The mom pushed and panted, gently giving counterpressure with one hand to the baby's head, helping it out slowly herself, with her eyes closed. The baby rotated to face her daddy, and he and his wife lifted the rest of the baby out and into the mother's arms. It was a beautiful birth, one where the parents did it all.

"Many times, our mere presence, and only our presence, is all that is necessary. This gives the client the confidence she needs. She may need us only to know that if there is a threat to the mother's or the baby's safety, she can depend on us to intervene with our special lifeguard skills."

CHOOSING A BACKUP HOSPITAL

A backup hospital within a twenty-minute drive of your home is an essential requirement for a safe home birth. Should a medical emergency arise during labor or the early postpartum period, you may need to transfer to the hospital without delay. Select your backup hospital during your pregnancy. Your caregiver will probably already have arrangements with one or more institutions in the area.

Cheri and Martin chose two backup hospitals, both about the same distance from their home. "If there was a problem during labor we decided to go to the hospital that had a reputation for progressive obstetric care," they explained. "If there was a problem with the baby, we planned to go to the high-risk center."

If possible, select a hospital supportive of your plans. That way, the staff will be far more helpful if a last-minute transfer is necessary. In many areas of the United States, your choice may be limited. You may not be able to find a hospital with supportive staff and may have to make do with what is available. Unfortunately, planning a safe home birth in America sometimes consists of making compromises.

The information in Chapter Seven, on choosing a hospital, also applies to selecting a backup hospital. You might want to read that chapter after reading this section.

When Is a Transfer Necessary?

At the end of this section is a list of reasons that may cause you to be transferred to a hospital. Life-threatening complications such as severe fetal distress, prolapsed cord, or maternal hemorrhage are comparatively rare. But they do sometimes occur and when they do, emergency transfer is mandatory.

More often than not, however, parents transfer for less severe complications. For example, the most common medical problems that developed in over 3,500 Arizona mothers planning to give birth at home attended by a lay midwife were premature rupture of membranes, premature onset of labor, and delayed onset of labor beyond forty-two weeks' gestation. In cases like this, there is usually no rush. You can go to the hospital at your leisure.

Whatever your reason, transfer will be less traumatic if you carefully plan for it in advance. Kathyleen, a mother who spent much time planning her home birth, recalls: "In my mind, I imagined everything that could go wrong and decided how I wanted each possibility handled. By the time of birth, my husband and midwife knew extensively what my concerns were and how I wanted to deal with possible problems."

The possibility of transfer is a good reason to make out a health-care checklist, expressing your preferences for care during labor, birth, and the early postpartum period.

The following are some of the major reasons mothers transfer from home to hospital. It is important that these conditions are diagnosed by a competent midwife or physician.

EMERGENCIES
Prolapsed cord. The umbilical cord precedes the baby's head in the birth canal, presenting a grave danger of fetal asphyxiation and death.

Bright red bleeding during pregnancy or labor. This is a possible sign that the placenta is overlying the cervix or is detached from the uterine wall. There is a serious danger of fetal death and maternal hemorrhage.

Baby is blue, limp, and not breathing. This presents a danger of fetal asphyxiation and death, and immediate resuscitation at home is imperative. However, the baby is usually transferred later for further care.

Baby's heart rate is low (under 100) or racing (180). Known as fetal distress, this presents the danger of inadequate oxygen, brain damage, and death.

Maternal hemorrhage after birth. This can involve either profuse bleeding or a continuous trickle of blood.

Other Reasons for Transfer

Prolonged rupture of membranes. There is a risk of infection after twenty-four hours. The caregiver may prefer keeping the mother at home and monitoring her for signs of infection.

Premature labor. Labor is considered premature if it begins three weeks or more before the due date.

Postmature labor. This refers to labor that begins more than three weeks past the due date.

Greenish or brownish amniotic fluid. This indicates that the baby has passed meconium and may or may not have continued fetal distress. (Meconium is the sticky greenish-black substance of the baby's first stool. It is sometimes passed in the uterus when the baby is distressed.)

Prolonged labor or lack of progress. Before transferring to the hospital you should try other methods to induce or enhance labor with your caregiver's approval. These include activities such as walking, lovemaking or nipple stimulation, and relaxation. (Both lovemaking with orgasm and nipple stimulation release the hormone oxytocin, which can trigger labor contractions if the cervix is ripe and the mother is ready to go into labor. This is certainly a more natural and enjoyable way to enhance labor than taking an oxytocic drug.)

Mother's feeling that she should be in a hospital. You may have an intuition that you need medical care in the hospital or that something isn't right. Pay attention to this intuition. Let your body be your guide. If you are more comfortable in a hospital, giving birth there will be a more positive experience.

Baby in the breech position. In this position, the baby's feet or buttocks—rather than the head—are first in the birth canal. This is usually, but not always, diagnosed prenatally.

Multiple pregnancy (twins, triplets, or more). This is usually, but not always, diagnosed prenatally, and risk increases with the number of babies.

Placenta does not deliver within one-half to one hour after birth.

Retained placenta fragments. These may have to be checked in the hospital.

Maternal tears that the caregiver is unable to repair at home.

Any other condition requiring medical treatment or observation.

HOME-BIRTH SUPPLIES

Did you ever wonder what all that boiling water in movies and television birth scenes was for? Most often, it's used for sterilizing scissors, cord clamps, or string to tie the umbilical cord. However, in all the home births I've attended, the only thing I've ever seen boiling water used for is tea and coffee.

You will need several supplies other than boiling water. Check the list that follows and then find out what your caregiver plans to bring and what you are expected to purchase.

You can obtain supplies from many drugstores, medical-supply houses, or a mail-order business specializing in childbirth supplies such as Naturpath. (Naturpath is located at 1410 N.W. 13th Street, Gainesville, Florida 32601; telephone 1-800-542-4784.)

FOR LABOR AND BIRTH:

- two sets of clean sheets, one set for birth and one set for afterward
- a waterproof pad or sheet to prevent staining the mattress (a shower curtain or large plastic tablecloth works fine)
- disposable absorbent pads (such as Chux by Johnson & Johnson or large diapers) to place beneath the mother
- clean towels
- clean washcloths for compresses
- one to two dozen sterile gauze pads (for perineal support as the baby is born)
- six to twelve pairs of disposable sterile gloves
- trash bags
- oil for massage (a new bottle of unopened vitamin E oil or olive oil is often recommended)
- umbilical-cord clamps
- a three-ounce bulb syringe (to suction mucus from the baby's mouth and nose)
- hot tea and honey and plenty of other liquids such as juice or bottled water
- food for those attending the birth
- a mirror so mother can watch the birth
- a large bowl to catch the placenta

FOR AFTER THE BIRTH:

- cotton balls and rubbing alcohol to cleanse the umbilical cord after it is cut
- receiving blankets for the newborn
- sanitary napkins (hospital size) and a sanitary belt
- two to three ounces of comfrey leaves and gauze (to apply to perineal tears or stitches). Comfrey is wonderful at promoting healing.

WHY IS THERE PREJUDICE AGAINST HOME BIRTH?

In some children's books or magazines, you'll find drawings that include an absurd element such as a dinosaur playing the flute. The object for the child is to pick out what's out of place. Being a consumer of obstetric care in America is a little like being that child: you must pick out the absurdities. And it's quite a task. There are probably more flute-playing dinosaurs in American childbirth than there are in the birth customs of just about every other nation in the world.

Throughout anthropological literature you'll find few things stranger than some of those associated with "typical" American birth—from routine perineal shaving to maternal–infant separation during the first hours after birth. We are so used to such things, we often fail to see how unnecessary—and often counterproductive—they are.

One of the strangest things about American birth is the widespread prejudice against home birth. Until the 1930s, the overwhelming majority of births in this country occurred at home, yet having a baby at home is still considered unconventional behavior here. As one home-birth practitioner puts it: "It is a comment on our times that we, who want childbirth to once again become an intimate family affair filled with the security of one's home and the love of one's family, are considered radicals."

Often parents are the ones to suffer from the prejudice against home birth. As childbirth educator and anthropologist Lester Hazell puts it: "If you have your baby at home, you will be going counter to the social trend. This means that you have to be braced against remarks if you tell people ahead of time you plan to do this. It also means that if anything goes wrong, you are in a position of having brought it on yourself and your baby. Our strange society will not hold it against you if your baby is palsied or his intelligence is stunted by too much anesthesia in the hospital, but if he is born at home with a birthmark or a clubfoot, the fault will be called yours!"

Home-birth parents also face the harassment of health professionals. Some doctors, for example, have been known to refer to home birth as "child abuse"—a statement as foolish as it is heinous. And there are some physicians who even refuse to provide prenatal care to a mother who intends to give birth at home with a midwife. (In my opinion, this is a form of malpractice far graver than that for which most physicians are sued.) There also are unfortunate cases of home-birth mothers who have had to be transferred to hospitals as a result of complications arising during the course of labor or the early postpartum period who have been treated with insensitivity by the hospital staff. For example, after her second birth, one Florida mother had a retained placenta (a complication having nothing to do with the place of birth). She was transferred from home to hospital. During her hospital stay, several nurses criticized her decision to give birth at home with comments such as "You must have been crazy to attempt a home birth!"

Fortunately, however, many health professionals who disagree with parents' choices to give birth at home or who don't approve of the home-birth practices of their peers recognize that parents and professionals have the right to choose the options that best suit them.

Many physicians feel home birth represents a giant step backwards. One reason for this is their experience with complications. Home birth is frightening to many physicians, midwives, and nurses who have been constantly surrounded by complications, some stemming from poor maternal health, others from obstetrical procedures. The daily confrontation with problems in the hospital reinforces the belief that birth is fraught with risks. Accordingly, the practitioner develops a fear or hesitancy of being away from technical equipment and staff that can help in emergencies. By contrast, home-birth practitioners, thanks to careful screening and the promotion of healthy prenatal habits, are surrounded by primarily normal births. Their view that home birth is safe is continually reinforced.

Another reason behind the opposition is simply economic. Home birth is less profitable for the practitioner, who may be stuck in a laboring woman's home for hours. While in the hospital, the physician can take care of other responsibilities, see other patients, or even attend to several labors at the same time. While this makes perfect sense to the physician, there is no reason it should influence your position.

Concern about malpractice also looms large in physician resistance to home birth. As one physician puts it, "I might be more supportive of lay midwives if my malpractice insurance wasn't $23,000." It is easy to understand his feeling. Today, in our litigious society, it is a risk to be a conventional obstetrician let alone one who bucks the established patterns of practice. The health-care consumer is largely to blame for the malpractice crisis because of the high numbers of unwarranted suits filed. At the same time, however, we might reflect on the fact that while obstetricians are frequently sued, rarely is a suit brought against a midwife. This could be partly because the midwife makes every effort to help the mother give birth the way she desires.

Another factor contributing to health professionals' resistance is what I have found to be a kind of hard-headed refusal to consider something beyond their immediate experience. As researchers Deborah A. Sullivan and Rose Weitz observe: "Physicians may present inappropriate evidence to bolster their opposition or may choose to ignore evidence that contradicts their preconceived ideas." They point out that physicians ignore home-birth studies as they have ignored evidence in favor of other health-care alternatives such as acupuncture.

LOOKING AHEAD

Planned childbirth at home attended by a midwife, physician, or physician-midwife team is the alternative of choice for an increasing number of parents. Home unquestionably provides a more comfortable, emotionally more positive birth environment for many parents. Studies to date have provided favorable information about childbirth at home, and it is my hope that more extensive studies will follow.

As more parents elect to give birth at home, home-birth services will become more widely available and home birth will become even more safe. Safety for mother and child could be greatly improved if more health-professional teams with emergency backup were widely distributed and more hospitals were willing to accept and accommodate parents in their community who choose to give birth at home.

Many home-birth parents—like home-birth midwives—are pioneers, particularly in areas where childbirth at home is not widely accepted. They must oppose the traditional health-care system. It takes courage to stand up against well-established medical policies (even when the policies are often based on emotional prejudice rather than on science). Some home-birth parents become childbirth activists, champions for change of unfair laws, inspiring others to follow their example.

The parents who give birth at home today are blazing the way for a safer, saner obstetrics to be available when it is our children's turn to experience the joys of giving birth their way.

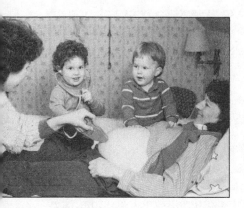

Birth in a Childbearing Center

BRIDGET'S FIRST CHILD WAS BORN in a hospital in the Los Angeles area. "There was nothing really bad about the birth," she recalls. "It was just impersonal. I felt like I was on an assembly line. But I was like a lot of women. I didn't know any better. Unless you've experienced something different, you may not even realize what you've missed. You may think hospital birth is the best there is."

The birth went well; mother and baby were healthy. But Bridget was disappointed, as she knew there was something missing. When she was pregnant again, she discovered an alternative. Her next child was born in the Marchbanks Alternative Childbearing Center in La Habra, California.

"I never imagined how different labor could be," Bridget said. "The birthing center was a personal, loving, and caring atmosphere. I was made to feel like I was the most special person on earth.

"There, having a baby wasn't just a woman's thing. The staff wanted both my husband, Tracy, and me to have the best experience. Dr. Marchbanks invited Tracy to be involved throughout. My family was also welcome. In addition to my husband, my mother, sister, sister-in-law, my aunt, and my grandma shared the birth. They physician remained with me the whole time during labor and after the birth. It made me feel special.

"We plan to have another child. And the birth will be at the childbearing center. There's just no comparing the two experiences."

A growing number of parents have discovered what Bridget has about childbirth in the birth center. This is especially true of mothers who have already had one or more babies in the hospital. They frequently opt to give birth to their next baby in a childbearing center either because they were dissatisfied with their hospital experience or are attracted to the idea of giving birth in a more homelike setting with flexible policies.

WHAT ARE CHILDBEARING CENTERS?

A childbearing center, also called a birthing, birth, or alternative-birth center, is a homelike facility outside a hospital setting for prenatal care, labor, birth, and the first few hours after birth. Many centers are called *free-standing* birth centers to indicate that they are physically, officially, and financially independent of a hospital.

About 50 percent of birthing centers are nonprofit organizations such as the cooperatively owned The Birth Place in Menlo Park, California. A percentage are owned by corporations. Some, like the Marchbanks Alternative Childbearing Center, are owned by private physicians or midwives. And an increasing number of centers are owned by hospitals, such as the Beverly Birth Center of Beverly, Massachusetts, run by Northshore Hospital and The Family Birth Center, an in-hospital center run by Providence Hospital in Southfield, Michigan.

Birth centers are modeled on the home, not the hospital. Perhaps the major factor distinguishing childbearing-center from hospital birth is, in the words of one midwife, "the feeling of giving birth at home away from home."

Though they vary from one center to another, birth-center policies are far more flexible than those in most hospitals. As The National Association for Childbearing Centers states: "Hospitals create policies to care for people who are sick, while free-standing birth centers design programs for healthy pregnant women."

In the birth center, during labor the mother is able to wear her own clothing, eat and drink, shower or bathe, walk around as she desires, and share her experience with her family and the guests of her choice. Most important, she, not the staff, is the center of the childbearing drama.

An Evolving Concept

Birth centers are relative newcomers to obstetric care. They evolved in the 1970s primarily to meet the needs of a growing number of parents who were dissatisfied with available maternity services, including traditional hospital delivery and home birth. According to Ruth Watson Lubic, General Director of the Maternity Center Association, the hospital health-care delivery system has failed for the most part to respond to the needs of childbearing families.

While home birth often meets the needs of the expectant parents, the lack of skilled, experienced home-birth practitioners in many areas left parents with either the traditional hospital, a home birth attended by a poorly trained midwife, or a do-it-yourself birth. Parents were actively seeking safe alternatives.

A few pioneer practitioners were willing to meet their clients' needs. For example, Dr. Howard E. Marchbanks, a pioneering southern California physician who attends hospital, childbearing-center, and home births, has been delivering babies in his own free-standing childbearing center since 1973. Dr. Marchbanks is committed to helping clients create the birth of their choice. He believes that the mother should have the option of choosing where her baby will be born. He even attended one couple's birth in a tent!

Other pioneers include Victor and Salee Berman, who created the first birth center in California and one of the first centers in the United States. Beginning with the desire to create a more humane experience for their clients within the hospital, they proposed a single room for labor, birth, and the postpartum period. Though such LDRP (labor, delivery, recovery, and postpartum) rooms are now common throughout the nation, at the time the Bermans proposed their idea, it was considered too unconventional. They therefore decided to create a birthplace within their OB/GYN office. This was the beginning of NACHIS, the Natural Childbirth Institute in Culver City, California.

Though a few practitioners like Dr. Marchbanks and the Bermans were providing a birth place for mothers in a homelike out-of-hospital environment, the Maternity Center Association (MCA) in New York City developed the first actual childbearing center to be accepted as a recognized part of the obstetric health-care system. The persons primarily responsible for this development were certified nurse-midwife Ruth Watson Lubic and the present director of the National Association for Childbearing Centers (NACC), Eunice Ernst, CNM.

MCA opened The Childbearing Center in September 1975 to provide safe obstetric care that was both sensitive to human needs and less expensive than hospital care. The center is located in a town house in Manhattan. MCA opted for opening the Childbearing Center in preference to creating a home delivery system for several reasons. First, home delivery was more expensive for the practitioner. Second, home birth has potential dangers not to the mother but to the practitioner traveling in New York City at odd hours of the night! As Ruth Lubic puts it: "Even in the mid-50's, safety of staff traveling through the city at all hours had become a problem for Maternity Center Association's home birth service which closed in 1958." MCA has since opened another birth center in New York, The Childbearing Center of Morris Heights in the Bronx.

As with most things representing change, birth centers have received mixed reactions ranging from enthusiastic applause to bitter condemnation. The latter stems primarily from physicians who are uncomfortable with client-centered obstetrics in a homelike atmosphere and who feel more comfortable in the clinical environment of the hospital. But, despite its initial bitter opposition by physicians, the Childbearing Center was opened. And it has provided the inspiration that has changed the face of childbirth forever.

Other free-standing childbearing centers opened throughout the United States within a few months. "We borrowed heavily from Ruth Lubic and the Maternity Center Association when we set up our birthing center here in Douglasville, Georgia," says obstetrician Dr. Richard B. Stewart. "They broke the ground for us." The Douglasville Birthing Center, opened in 1976, was the first in-hospital birth center in Georgia.

More childbearing centers are opening throughout the United States in response to the needs of expectant parents. However, one-third or more of those that open soon close their doors. There are a couple of reasons for this: many birth centers are opened by one or two physicians or midwives who lack the business skills to keep them running, and some centers simply don't meet the clients' needs for which these unique facilities were originally designed—namely, a homelike environment where the mother can receive noninterventive midwifery care. A few are more like mini-hospitals than birth centers. One physician who opened a childbearing center that remained in business only about a year said he opened it only to keep up with the competition. Nevertheless, there are currently well over 250 childbearing centers scattered throughout the United States, and there is every reason to believe they will continue to evolve and their numbers grow.

The Place

One family physician described his vision of the ideal childbearing center to me:

"An old house with three or four small separate living areas, each with its own kitchenette and bathroom with both shower and tub. Each living area should also have a separate musical facility so individual families could play the music of their choice during labor. The furnishings should include antiques or modern furniture made in the old style, an antique rocking chair for the mother to use during labor, and lots of braided rugs for that homey feeling.

"For the birthing bed, an 800-thousand-dollar piece of equipment such as those in some hospital birthing rooms is hardly necessary. A comfortable double or queen-sized bed with lots of pillows will suffice.

"The house should be staffed with full-time midwives. It matters little whether they are certified nurse-wives or lay midwives as long as they are well-trained and competent.

"Of course, the center should have a large yard with a play area for other children and a large playroom with lots of toys that can be used in inclement weather. This way, children attending births won't have to be sequestered in one area throughout labor.

"To keep everything centrally located, all prenatal care should take place in offices out of sight and sound in a basement or first floor.

"There is no reason centers like this can't exist right on the hospital grounds as well as independent of hospitals."

Few of the childbearing centers are quite as beautiful as this physician's description. Most do not have entire living areas for each family, but birthing rooms only. Most do not have a yard where children can play. However, many centers—whether in Victorian homes or modern single-story buildings—attempt to come as close as they can to this vision.

Childbearing centers are usually renovated homes, though an increasing number are being created in professional office space and one center is in an apartment high-rise. The majority are independent of hospitals.

The best birth centers have two or more private, attractively decorated birth rooms. These are generally equipped with either an ordinary double bed (rather than a narrow hospital-sized bed) or a special birthing bed designed to facilitate obstetric care during labor and delivery. Cots or pullout couches are usually available for the mother's guests.

Many childbearing centers also have kitchen facilities the parents and those attending the birth can use. Some families bring their own food and drinks and prepare their own meals. By contrast, in the Family Birthing Center in Upland, California, owned by Dr. Michael Rosenthal, the new parents can order a gourmet meal to be delivered!

In addition, many birth centers have a family room; examining rooms; a Jacuzzi, spa, or oversized tub for the mother's use during labor; a classroom; a room with toys where siblings can play; and a lending library.

Examples of Childbearing Centers

Approximately five thousand babies have been born since 1973 in the Marchbanks Alternative Childbearing Center in La Habra, California. Managed by Barbara Mason, a childbirth educator whose radiant enthusiasm inspires confidence in the parents' ability to give birth naturally, this center has two small but beautiful birthing rooms in addition to examining rooms, a waiting room, and an office area. I had the opportunity to observe the birth of a baby girl there one weekend when I was in the area to conduct workshops. The room where the birth took place had a double bed and beautiful blue walls painted with clouds through which shone the rays of the sun. It was an appropriate and dramatic motif for a birthing room.

The midwife, Lorri Walker, R.N., knelt at the foot of the bed while catching the baby. As the baby's head was being born, Lorri gently massaged the perineum (the part of the pelvic region between the vagina and anus) so the mother would not tear. Then she guided the mother's hands to take the baby under the arms and complete her own birth. The beautiful, natural birth took place in a room suffused with a sense of peace as the father held his wife closely.

Each room at this center is equipped with a soft cotton rope, hanging from the ceiling like a vine. Many mothers find it helpful to hang on the rope while pushing. "It's amazing how this can facilitate the descent of a baby during a difficult second stage," says Barbara Mason.

The Birth Center in Houston, Texas, owned and operated by certified nurse-midwife Pat Jones, has a similar homelike setting. It is in a two-story Victorian home with two birthing rooms. Each room has a large closet where medical equipment is stored. The rooms are attractively decorated to look like home bedrooms. The first floor includes an office for prenatal exams, a large living room, and an eat-in kitchen clients may use at their convenience.

FamilyBorn, an alternative-birth center owned and operated by certified nurse-midwife Elizabeth Clifton about an hour-and-fifteen-minute drive from St. Louis, in Perryville, Missouri, is a remodeled home. In addition to an office, a kitchen, and bathrooms, the center includes a family room, a birth room with a spa where the mother can labor and give birth if she wishes, a large old-fashioned bed, and a wardrobe with medical equipment. Clifton points out that at FamilyBorn most women don't use the bed to give birth. The majority feel more comfortable giving birth squatting on the floor over a sterile pad.

Jackson Memorial Hospital in Miami, Florida sponsors a unique free-standing childbearing center. Jackson Memorial is a tertiary facility (a hospital that provides care for high-risk clients who require the most sophisticated type of medical and technical intervention; full-time specialists and the most modern equipment are available). The Birth Center of Jackson was developed as a lower-cost alternative to traditional hospital care for low-risk childbearing families.

The center is located on the tenth floor of a high-rise building that also has offices, hotel rooms, and apartments. It consists of six large bedrooms, each with an adjoining private bath; two examination rooms; an education room; a waiting room; and offices. The Birth Center is staffed by certified nurse-midwives, a registered nurse, licensed practical nurses, and secretarial staff. The family stays together throughout labor and birth. Mothers are encouraged to walk around as they please and to eat and drink as needed.

Some births centers are more flexible than others and will accept a broader range of clients. All, however, are committed to providing safe alternative obstetric care outside the hospital setting. All provide settings more conducive than the conventional hospital to a spontaneous reaction to labor. For this reason, they offer a more positive birth experience for mother, father, and baby.

The Health Care

The care available at most childbearing centers is usually based on the view that birth is a normal, natural event. In the center, the mother and her mate have the right to choose how she will give birth and actively participate in the childbearing process. As Barbara Mason of the Marchbanks Alternative Childbearing Center puts it: "Here, we celebrate pregnancy and wellness. We want to get the message out that the mother's body functions without medical intervention in the overwhelming majority of cases."

Speaking about a childbearing center in Menlo Park, California, Pamela S. Eakins, PhD, of Stanford University, expresses a similar idea: "The Birth Place views childbirth as a physical, emotional, social, and spiritual rite of passage for mother and baby. Only secondarily is childbirth seen as a medical event."

Dr. Michael Rosenthal of the Family Birth Center in Upland, California, says: "We take the term 'non-intervention' in a very literal sense. It often means that women give birth without me using my hands."

The childbearing-center philosophy emphasizes taking part in one's own maternity care. For example, at the Marchbanks Alternative Childbearing Center, mothers who so wish are taught to test their own urine and record their weight at appointments. Fathers are shown the cervix and are taught how to do abdominal palpations (to feel the fetal outline) and how to time the duration and length of contractions.

The health care offered during pregnancy, labor, and the postpartum period varies somewhat from one birth center to another. Most, however, offer the following health care throughout the entire childbearing season.

Prenatal care. The majority of centers offer prenatal care as well as care during labor. However, a few centers provide health care only for labor, delivery, and the first hours postpartum. In this case, the mother receives her prenatal care elsewhere, usually with the midwife or physician who staffs the center.

Care during labor. In the best childbearing centers, the mother receives warm, personalized care. Nursing or midwifery care is almost always provided on a one-to-one basis.

A good birth center should have the ability to initiate emergency procedures in life-threatening situations and have a backup hospital nearby with a system for rapid transport.

In some birthing centers, pain medication such as Demerol is available should the mother request it. In others, the mother is transferred to a nearby hospital if the need for pain medication arises. Bear in mind that the need for medication is significantly decreased in the relaxing environment of the alternative-childbearing center. Carla Reinke, past executive director of the Birthplace, a free-standing nonprofit childbearing center in Seattle, Washington, says that at the Birthplace, "medication for pain relief during normal labor was virtually nonexistent, probably due to the education, motivation, and support provided women in labor."

The American Public Health Association's "Guidelines for Licensing and Regulating Birth Centers" recommend that labor not be stimulated or augmented with chemical agents such as Pitocin in the birth-center setting. However, Pitocin and other drugs are used in a few birth centers. For example, oxytocic drugs, as well as intravenous feeding, sedatives, and narcotics, are all available at the Alternative Birth Center in Jacksonville, Florida. Other stimulants to labor that are used in some birth centers include herbal preparations and acupuncture.

Creating a positive emotional climate and meeting the mother's emotional needs will greatly increase her chances of having a safe, positive birth experience, because the physical process of labor is readily influenced by the mother's emotions. This cannot be stressed enough. In my opinion, the major reason that childbearing-center care leaves parents with a far more positive perception of the birth experience than traditional hospital care is because the birth center is conducive toward eliciting the laboring mind response. When the mother is able to fully yield to the changes this response entails, her labor is more likely to progress more efficiently.

Myrtle Hosford, past coordinator of the Maternity Center Association in New York City, says: "It is not enough to merely monitor labor and safeguard its course. Creating a physical and emotional atmosphere in which sensitivity to needs and intimacy prevail may be more important to the process of labor and its ultimate outcome than any other single factor."

Postpartum care. Mother and baby usually remain in the center for twelve to twenty-four hours, then return home. Some centers request that she return within a few days after discharge for a brief checkup. A few centers arrange for a nurse or midwife to visit the mother in her home a few days after birth.

Additional services. Many birthing centers also offer childbirth classes, new-parents' support groups, well-child care, and women's health care.

The Care Providers

In childbearing centers, maternity care is provided by a variety of health professionals: certified nurse-midwives, obstetricians, family physicians, a midwife-physician team, and lay midwives. However, in the majority of childbearing centers certified nurse-midwives provide this care.

Many centers are staffed by one or two midwives with no additional staff. For instance, certified nurse-midwife Elizabeth Clifton and her assistant comprise the entire staff at FamilyBorn Birth Center in Perryville, Missouri. In addition to a busy home-birth practice, Elizabeth Clifton handles all the births taking place in the two attractively furnished rooms of her center. Other centers include a backup physician, such as the Marchbanks Alternative Childbearing Center in La Habra, California, which is staffed by a family physician in addition to a midwife.

A growing number of centers are owned and operated by obstetricians. Dr. Michael Rosenthal, owner of the Family Birthing Center in Upland, California, has a staff consisting of around-the-clock registered nurses, two certified nurse-midwives, and administrative personnel. In addition, childbirth educators teach classes in the center and a lactation consultant is available to give breast-feeding information and help.

In The Birth Place, a nonprofit organization in Menlo Park, California in a three-bedroom renovated house, several community-health professionals including an obstetrician, family physicians, and certified nurse-midwives attend women in labor. Obstetric nurses and trained assistants are on call twenty-four hours a day.

A few centers also employ childbirth assistants. For example, the Washington Birthing Center in Fremont, California, located directly across the street from Washington Township Hospital, employs childbirth assistants as full-time staff members twenty-four hours a day. There, everyone works as a team to support the mother and her family. Gail Fiock, a childbirth assistant at the center, says, "In addition to giving labor support, our duties include care of the linen, taking vital signs, cleaning and restocking the birthing rooms, cooking for mothers and their families as needed, and paperwork."

The advantage of an on-staff childbirth assistant is additional

labor support for the mother, which has been associated with reduced complications and shorter labors. Ideally, the mother should
be able to choose her own labor-support person.

Lay midwives also practice in a few childbearing centers. Even
in states where lay midwifery is not legally recognized, a few
maverick physicians will permit a skilled lay midwife to give prenatal care and deliver babies. However, given the legal standing of lay
midwifery, this fact is usually not advertised.

SAFETY OF CHILDBEARING CENTERS

A recent nationwide study published in the *New England Journal of
Medicine*, the "National Birth Center Study," shows that free-
standing birth centers provide a safe alternative to hospital birth
for healthy women with normal pregnancies. Researchers analyzed
the experiences of 11,814 laboring women at eighty-four free-
standing birth centers. The mothers were at lower-than-average
risk of a poor outcome of pregnancy. The study states: "Researchers found that the infant-mortality rate was as low as that
found in studies of hospitals with similar low-risk mothers. Meanwhile, there was a higher degree of personal satisfaction among
women who gave birth in childbearing centers."

Several factors contribute to the safety of chilbearing-center
birth.

- Prenatal screening is done to help identify problems that
  could predispose the mother to complications during labor.
- The birth center is staffed by skilled, experienced midwives
  or physicians.
- Equipment to handle medical emergencies is readily available.
- The mother receives individual care throughout labor.
- Most centers have a cooperative relationship with a nearby
  hospital in case a last-minute transfer is necessary. A system
  for rapid transport to the nearby hospital is also available.

A study of randomly selected mothers who chose childbearing-
center and home birth revealed that the majority felt in-hospital
birth was as risky or more risky than birth out of the hospital. The

risks they mentioned include infection, mother–infant separation, induced labor, surgical birth, and being pressured into accepting excessive interventions, including drugs.

The major reason mothers choose a childbearing center in preference to home birth is safety. However, unless the center is closer to a hospital than the mother's home, home birth is probably just as safe *providing the mother is effectively screened for risk and the birth is attended by an experienced midwife or physician with medical equipment.*

The mother who plans a childbearing-center birth should get good prenatal care and observe healthy habits throughout pregnancy. In her practice in southern California, Lynn Amin, CNM, has observed, "Clients who don't follow a good diet, are overweight, and who aren't active are the ones most likely to have complications and be transferred to the hospital."

As I've mentioned, in most childbearing centers the expectant mother is carefully screened to ensure that her chances of a normal, healthy birth are good. Of course, this doesn't rule out all possibilities of complications. Unusual complications do occasionally arise. Some problems such as placental abruption (the placenta detaching from the uterine wall) are better handled in a hospital. A list of conditions that can cause transfer from a childbearing center can be found on page 157.

WHO GIVES BIRTH IN CHILDBEARING CENTERS?

Childbearing centers vary in their criteria for accepting clients. In 1979, The American Public Health Association (APHA) adopted a set of guidelines for licensing and regulating birth centers, emphasizing that only mothers with normal, uncomplicated pregnancies who were expected to have uncomplicated labors should be accepted as clients.

Complications preventing mothers from giving birth in childbearing centers are similar to those ruling out home birth. These include maternal illness such as diabetes, chronic hypertension, complications of labor such as breech position, and premature labor.

However, as I mentioned in Chapter Two, "low risk" is a relative term. Caregivers have different criteria for deciding just what constitutes low risk. The purpose of risk-screening is to ensure the safety of mother and baby. Each mother, I believe, should be assessed on an individual basis.

Unfortunately, in many centers, policies for risk assessment have become rigid. Many focus more on the policy than on the person. Some caregivers will not accept perfectly healthy clients simply because they feel the clients belong in an arbitrarily defined "high-risk" category. For example, many centers will not accept clients over thirty-five or under nineteen years of age or women who are planning a vaginal birth after a cesarean. Providing the mother's health is normal and there are no complications in her pregnancy, the mother over thirty-five or the woman who is planning a VBAC has just as much of a chance of a safe, positive birth as anyone else. When childbearing centers use arbitrary risk-screening criteria, they often exclude perfectly healthy mothers.

Strict policies for accepting clients or transferring clients to hospitals are not always the fault of the childbearing center. Often, as Eunice Ernst puts it, "this is an example of demonstrating the art of compromise. In some areas, if it weren't for adopting certain policies, the childbearing center would never have been opened."

As Dr. Richard B. Stewart of the Douglas Birthing Center, an in-hospital childbearing center in Douglas General Hospital in Douglasville, Georgia, complains: "The medical community can be like a watchdog in making sure that you transfer every little complication. For example, if the mother loses 475 cc of blood postpartum, she may not be in any trouble or need anything. However, she fits the criterion for postpartum hemorrhage, which is a loss of greater than 450 cc, and therefore has to be transferred. To have the medical community looking over your shoulder with such criticism and to have to observe every little criterion to the letter is a pain in the butt."

The VBAC mother and others with special needs may benefit from the positive emotional climate of the childbearing center. Therefore, unless there are real medical complications during her present pregnancy, the option of childbearing-center birth should be open to her.

Dr. Michael Rosenthal of the Family Birthing Center says, "Risk assessment is the most important thing in deciding who you are going to accept as a client." However, his concept of low risk is much broader than that of most physicians and midwives who run birthing centers. His birth-center clients range in age from sixteen to forty-three, and he readily accepts VBAC mothers—even those who have had multiple cesareans. Between 1985 and 1990, 154 VBAC mothers have given birth in the Family Birthing Center without complications.

Childbearing centers that are in very close proximity to hospitals, however, can take clients considered to be at greater risk. The Family Birthing Center is only 150 yards from a hospital. "This allows us to be more flexible about our clients than we might be if we were five miles from a hospital," Dr. Rosenthal points out. Many birthing centers will not accept clients in labor who are more than two weeks preterm. Dr. Rosenthal, on the other hand, will accept clients four and even five weeks preterm. "If a baby needs time in an intensive-care nursery," he says, "we simply walk the baby across the street to the hospital. Should an emergency requiring a cesarean section arise, a client can be transferred to the hospital and brought into surgery in less time than many hospitals can set up for surgical birth."

Ironically, while childbearing centers that are very close to hospitals can safely accept clients at greater risk of a complicated labor, birth centers owned and operated by hospitals often have the strictest screening criteria of all due to rigid hospital policy.

CONDITIONS EXCLUDING THE USE OF THE CHILDBEARING CENTER

Childbearing centers vary in their criteria for accepting clients. Some birth centers will not accept a woman who has one of the following conditions.

Conditions relating to past pregnancies and births

- Grandmultiparity (seven or more previous births; in some birth centers, the mother with three previous births is considered a grandmultipara)
- Previous cesarean section
- Previous premature birth (usually two or more previous premature births)
- Rh sensitization
- Incompetent cervix (that is, the cervix dilates prior to labor's onset)

- Previous birth to infant with severe congenital abnormality, such as cerebral palsy
- Previous difficult vaginal delivery
- Previous stillbirth
- History of three or more miscarriages
- History of postpartum hemorrhage

Current medical conditions

- Chronic hypertension
- Maternal illness such as diabetes mellitus, epilepsy, renal disease, thyroid disease, heart disease, pulmonary disease, sickle-cell disease, and so forth.
- Severe obesity
- Drug addiction and alcohol abuse

Conditions of the current pregnancy

- Excessive or inadequate weight gain
- Preeclampsia
- Significant vaginal bleeding
- Anemia
- Multiple pregnancy
- Premature labor (occurring prior to thirty-seven weeks' gestation)
- Postmature labor (occurring after forty-two weeks' gestation)
- Malpresentation (fetus in other than the vertex position)
- Prolonged rupture of membranes (longer than twenty-four hours without labor's onset)
- Intrauterine growth retardation
- Polyhydramnios or oligohydramnios (too much or too little amniotic fluid)
- Active herpes infection at the time of labor
- Syphilis
- Infectious disease such as toxoplasmosis or rubella
- Placenta previa (placenta is obstructing the cervical opening)
- Placental abruption

- Other diseases of pregnancy, such as hyperemisis gravi-
  darum (severe persistent vomiting)
- Any other condition for which hospitalization may be
  advisable

THE ADVANTAGES OF CHILDBEARING-CENTER BIRTH

"After my first birth in the hospital I felt drained and exhausted,"
says an Oregon mother quoted by the National Association of
Childbearing Centers. "I couldn't get any rest there for three days.
At the Birth Center I delivered at ten A.M. and was sitting on my
front porch rocking my baby at five P.M. I felt exhilarated and ter-
rific. What a difference the care makes."

The childbearing center is the ideal alternative for a growing
number of parents throughout the world for several reasons.

*The childbearing center is specifically associated only with preg-
nancy and birth.* Many women feel more comfortable in the health-
oriented setting of the childbearing center. Unlike hospitals, these
centers are not illness-oriented, and they, therefore provide a welcome alternative to the hospital setting. As Dr. Herbert Ratner, former health commissioner for Oak Park, Illinois, and a retired professor at Loyola University in Chicago puts it: "Anything is better
than a hospital. Hospitals are for sick people; being pregnant is not
a disease."

The health care provided at most birth centers stems from a
foundation of noninterventive obstetric care. Though expert medical care is available and, at most birth centers, medical equipment is
close at hand should it be necessary, the emphasis is on the nor-
mality of labor.

*The childbearing center presents a welcome alternative for parents
who are not comfortable with home birth yet don't want to give birth
in a hospital.* Lynn Amin, a certified nurse-midwife who attends
births both at home and in her childbearing center in Riverside,
California, admits, "My heart is with home birth." However, she
opened a beautiful birthing center with a homelike environment
because many of her clients were uncomfortable giving birth in

their own homes. "Home birth is not widely accepted in the United States," she points out. "A lot of women, especially first-time mothers, are afraid to give birth at home. In this culture, mothers are accustomed to going somewhere to have their babies. The childbearing center is becoming the place to go." She adds, "If they come here, I clean up. If I go to their house, they clean up!"

In many cases, the mother *feels* more comfortable and safer in the birthing center. Feeling more secure enables many women to better surrender to labor and therefore to labor more efficiently.

Childbearing centers offer personalized obstetric care. Practitioners in most birth centers will individualize the care they provide to meet the parents' desires providing nothing compromises the health of mother or baby.

"We invite parents to ask questions and express their preferences," says Barbara Mason. "There are almost no rules here that can't be broken to meet a mother's or family's needs."

In most childbearing centers, the clients are able to meet the entire staff before the birth. "We all become friends," says Lynn Amin. At her birth center, the expectant parents meet her backup physician and any of the nurses who may be attending. This isn't the case at all childbearing centers, however. A few are staffed by nurses around the clock and clients rarely are able to meet them all even though they visit the birth center for prenatal appointments.

In the childbearing center, the mother has a reduced chance of a cesarean section. The noninterventive care available in childbearing centers dramatically decreases the mother's chance of an unnecessary cesarean. The National Birth Center Study showed that the cesarean rate of nearly twelve thousand mothers who gave birth in childbearing centers was 4.4 percent, whereas the United States national average cesarean rate is a full 25 percent. Of course, the national rate includes mothers at high risk, while most birth centers serve only low-risk clients. Nevertheless, even the low-risk mother is at increased risk of cesarean surgery as a result of the medical intervention common in traditional hospitals.

For example, a study compared a matched group of 250 low-risk mothers delivering in Jackson Memorial Hospital in Miami, Florida with a matched group of mothers giving birth at the Birth Center of Jackson, located across the street. The cesarean rate among the birth-center mothers was 6 percent—less than half that for mothers in the hospital (14 percent). This has been found true for other childbearing centers as well.

The childbearing center offers obstetric care at a significantly lower cost than the traditional hospital. Cost of prenatal care and birth in childbearing centers varies depending on the area. Health care in birth centers is covered by most major medical insurance policies, including, in most states, Medicaid and Champus (Civilian Health and Medical Program of the Uniformed Services). Since not all insurance companies cover home birth, this makes the birth center more attractive to many parents.

Additionally, childbearing-center birth has many of the same advantages as home birth. These include greater control of the birth experience, the mother's freedom to do whatever she wants during labor, the parents' freedom to invite whomever they want to their birth, the ability to avoid unnecessary medical intervention, and the ability to labor in a comfortable, nonclinical setting.

Bear in mind not all of these benefits are available in every birth center. Some centers have rigid policies and less-than-ideal obstetric care. However, the benefits in this section do apply to the majority of birth centers.

BENEFITS OF CHILDBEARING-CENTER BIRTH

The following benefits are associated with giving birth in childbearing centers.

- Absence of restrictive policies
- Noninterventive obstetric care
- The mother's ability to invite the guests of her choice
- Reduced chance of a cesarean section
- Reduced need for pain-relief medication
- The freedom to give birth in the position of choice
- The freedom to eat and drink during labor
- The ability to labor and give birth in a homelike environment associated with childbirth, not with illness

- Reduced cost in comparison with hospital birth
- A more positive birth experience

DISADVANTAGES OF CHILDBEARING CENTERS

Though childbearing centers offer many benefits to a growing number of families, there are a few disadvantages. These vary with the individual center, the location, and the health care available.

- Although childbearing centers have more flexible policies than hospitals, the mother is still not on her own turf, as she would be at home.
- Rigid screening criteria often eliminate the perfectly healthy mother (such as the VBAC mother, the woman over thirty-five, or the mother with prolonged ruptured membranes).
- Many childbearing centers have rigid rules about transferring mothers to hospitals for conditions that could just as well be handled in the center, such as prolonged labor and ruptured membranes.

Another potential disadvantage is that as childbearing centers become increasingly popular and physicians opt for giving care in centers to keep up with the competition, the childbearing center is in danger of becoming more like a hospital than a home. This already describes many centers where rigid policies and protocol rule.

Dr. Michael Rosenthal points out: "Childbearing centers owned by obstetricians frequently fail because the doctors insist on practicing obstetrics rather than midwifery." This means that rather than offering the noninterventive care that makes birth centers unique, the physician gives the intervention-oriented obstetric care for which thousands of parents are leaving hospitals.

CHOOSING A CHILDBEARING CENTER

In most areas, your choice of childbearing centers will be limited to the center closest to your home. However, in some cities you may have several choices. For example, there are more childbearing centers in the Los Angeles area than in all of New England! In northern

New Hampshire, where I live, there are, unfortunately, no child-bearing centers.

To find a childbearing center, check the yellow pages. Ask a childbirth educator if there are any centers within a reasonable drive to your home. You can also contact the National Association of Childbearing Centers (NACC) at 215-234-8068 or write RFD 1, Perkiomenville, Pennsylvania 18074 and ask for a list of childbirth centers. Enclose a self-addressed stamped envelope. Here are some suggestions to make sure the birth center you choose is right for you.

Visit the childbearing center. Meet and talk with the staff; they should welcome you. The ideal childbearing center should be a homelike environment where you feel that you—not the staff—are the center of the childbearing drama.

Learn about the center's policies. Do they agree with your birth plans? Most centers have flexible policies. Within reason, you can do just about anything you want. However, as previously noted, restrictive policies and a clinical-looking environment make a few childbearing centers more like mini-hospitals than home.

Find out about the childbearing center's transfer criteria. For what reasons are most mothers transferred to hospitals? Some centers are more stringent about transfer regulations than others.

Find out how close the birth center is to a hospital in case transfer is necessary. Visit the hospital to become familiar with its environment and policies.

Find out what maternity care is available at the center. Are you given prenatal care? Postpartum care?

When you have selected a childbearing center, discuss your birth plans with your caregiver. For more on the relationship between your caregiver and the childbearing center, see Chapter Three.

Transfer to a Hospital

As previously noted, a mother may be transferred from childbearing center to hospital for a variety of reasons, including slow progress during labor, prolonged first- or second-stage labor, fetal distress, maternal hemorrhage, and other complications. A baby may be transferred if medical complications such as breathing difficulty make immediate pediatric attention necessary.

One woman in six of the 11,814 in the National Birth Center

Study was transferred to the hospital. This, in my opinion, is a very high rate of transfer, and it is far higher than the transfer rates in some centers. For example, only one in twenty at the Marchbanks Alternative Childbearing Center was transferred, the major reason being maternal exhaustion after a prolonged labor. Similarly, at the Baltimore Birth Center in Maryland (staffed by nurse-midwives) only about 7 percent were transferred; there, the major reason was lack of progress in labor, and the suggestion to go to the hospital was most often made by an exhausted mother after a long labor. "Transfer is always a joint decision between the mother and her midwife," says Ann Sober, R.N., who manages the center. Generally speaking, the rate of transfer in hospital-owned centers is higher than in free-standing childbearing centers.

Medical complications requiring hospital attention sometimes make transfer necessary. For example, one mother at the Family Birth Center in Upland, California had a prolapsed cord (a grave complication in which the umbilical cord precedes the baby in the birth canal, cutting off the baby's oxygen). She was transferred to the hospital across the street, where the baby was born healthy through an emergency cesarean section.

Some centers require transfer to the hospital if the mother requests pain-relief medication or any kind of medical intervention, such as the use of intravenous feeding for dehydration or the use of Pitocin to augment contractions. The health professionals running the Childbearing Center in New York City state: "Pitocin is never used to induce or stimulate labor in the setting, nor are forceps ever used. The setting is appropriate for midwifery management, but . . . an indication for obstetric management is an indication for transfer." Other centers, such as the Birth Center of Jackson in Miami, Florida, provide pain-relief medication and intravenous therapy as needed right in the center.

While obstetric intervention may be a good reason to shift location to the hospital, in my opinion, many mothers are transferred unnecessarily. For example, a major reason for transfer is prolonged labor. However, provided that the mother isn't exhausted and the fetal heart tones are normal, she can try a variety of methods to get labor going again—including guided imagery (particularly "The Opening Flower" and "Imagining the Birth" exercises), walking around, showering, bathing, nipple stimulation, lovemaking, or simply resting. If none of these methods work, transfer may be indicated.

Several studies have shown so-called arrested labor to be another major reason for transfer. In this condition, the cervix does not dilate for two or more hours or simply dilates slowly. Sometimes this is a genuine complication caused by any of a variety of factors such as fetal malposition, cephalopelvic disproportion (the head is thought to be too large for the maternal pelvis), and prior cervical surgery. However, in other cases, the cervix simply dilates slowly. Labor may stop for several hours and still be perfectly normal. Providing the mother and the baby are healthy, transfer is not essential.

In some birth centers, mothers are transferred even for prolonged early labor (that is, before the cervix is four to five centimeters dilated). However, it is perfectly normal for a mother to be in latent labor with on-and-off contractions for two days or more. Rather than be transferred to the hospital, she can simply go home until her labor becomes more active.

Yet another unnecessary reason for transfer is rupture of membranes (the "waters" breaking) for more than twenty-four hours or, in some childbearing centers, more than twelve hours without progress in labor. The mother with ruptured membranes who is not in labor is often taken to the hospital to have labor induced or augmented to avoid the risk of infection. For example, Emily, a New Jersey mother of two, wanted to give birth to her first child in a birth center. However, her membranes ruptured and the baby was not born within twenty-four hours, so she was transferred to a hospital. The experience was so disappointing to her she decided to give birth to her second child at home.

Alternatively, the mother can remain in the center and be monitored for signs of infection. "If the mother's membranes rupture and she isn't having contractions," says Barbara Mason of the Marchbanks Alternative Childbearing Center, "we ask her to take her temperature every two or three hours. We don't do any vaginal exams, which can greatly increase the chance of infection. If the mother has no signs of infection, there is no reason she should be transferred to the hospital."

There is little doubt that the transfer rates at many childbearing centers could be significantly reduced. However, mothers who are transferred—for whatever reason—often are still glad they chose the childbearing center. Many express appreciation for the care they received in the center up to the time of and during the transfer.

CONDITIONS FOR WHICH MOTHERS MAY BE TRANSFERRED FROM BIRTH CENTER TO HOSPITAL

Childbearing centers vary in their transfer criteria. Many will transfer mothers only for the more severe of the following conditions.

- Development of hypertension
- Malpresentation (baby in other than vertex position)
- Prolonged rupture of membranes
- Premature labor
- Any problem requiring forceps delivery or cesarean
- Mother requesting pain-relief medication or anesthesia or requiring use of intravenous feeding or Pitocin augmentation of labor
- Meconium staining of the amniotic fluid
- Abnormal fetal heart rate or pattern
- Lack of progress in labor
- Prolonged labor
- Cephalopelvic disproportion
- Prolapsed cord
- Placental abruption
- Placenta previa
- Maternal fever (greater than 100.4 degrees F)
- Extensive lacerations
- Retained placenta
- Maternal bleeding
- Any other condition requiring medical treatment or observation

CONDITIONS FOR WHICH A NEWBORN MAY BE TRANSFERRED FROM BIRTH CENTER TO HOSPITAL

After birth, the baby may be transferred from the childbearing center to the hospital for any of the following reasons.

- Apgar score of less than 7 at five minutes after birth
- Abnormal vital signs
- Signs of pre- or postmaturity
- A congenital abnormality
- Respiratory distress
- Low birth weight, jaundice, or any other condition requiring medical treatment or observation

LOOKING AHEAD

The primary feature that makes childbearing centers special—and more attractive than hospitals to an increasing population—is that the childbearing-center care is modeled on home birth.

I hope that in the future we will see more childbearing centers for high- as well as low-risk mothers. These women are just as much in need of the emotionally positive climate the childbearing center offers as everyone else. In fact, given their greater chance of developing complications, they are even more in need of a peaceful, homelike setting.

In the birth center, the emotional tension of the hospital—where problems are anticipated—is absent. The setting is not only relaxing but is also focused on life and on the parents. The care is based on women's needs, not on medical protocol. As Dr. Rosenthal puts it: "There is more touch than technology."

The sense of frustration, of being cheated out of participating in one of life's most precious experiences, and feelings of failure so common among mothers who give birth in traditional hospitals are rare among birth-center mothers. Women leave centers with a feeling of satisfaction. The overwhelming majority of mothers (98.8 percent) included in the National Birth Center Study said they would recommend birth centers to their friends, and 94 percent said they would use the center during future pregnancies. Even among the mothers who were transferred to hospitals, 96.9 percent said they would recommend childbearing centers to friends.

In childbearing centers women are *giving birth*, not having their babies *delivered*. It is for this reason I believe that the future of childbirth in the United States and in many other nations throughout the world will be in childbearing centers.

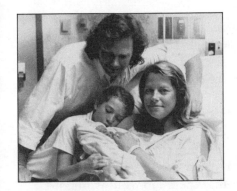

Hospital Birth

BEV, A MOTHER OF TWO, GAVE birth in a hospital whose staff was wholly committed to supporting her birth plans. She recalls: "The birthing room was filled with warmth, smiles, and wonder. My husband, Greg, and I had the kind of childbirth experience we wanted: family-oriented, no routine electronic monitoring, no episiotomy—soft lights and a warm, inviting room with regular old beds. Our wishes were respected and our four-year-old son, Joshua, was welcome to share in the joy and the miracle of birth.

"My labor went quickly. Contractions were intense but controllable with no special breathing needed. Second stage lasted only fifteen minutes. As the baby was born, Joshua sat on my midwife's lap at the edge of the bed, wide-eyed. The physician dimmed the lights. I could feel myself opening, stretching wider and wider with an intense burning feeling. Short quick breaths helped me relax and my body eased the baby out. The beautiful baby I longed to greet was placed on my belly. Together, our family welcomed seven-pound, twelve-ounce, twenty-one-inch Heather Elizabeth into a sensitive, gentle, intimate world."

Hospital birth can be a wonderful, rewarding event, a memory to be forever cherished. Or it can be a negative experience. One can no more make blanket statements about giving birth in hospitals than one can make generalizations about eating in restaurants. Some places leave you with fond memories; others make you wish you had never walked in the door.

Each hospital must be assessed individually. This chapter will give you some guidelines to help you make a wise choice.

HOSPITAL MATERNITY CARE IS CHANGING

Happily, a more humanized maternity care is evolving in many hospitals throughout the United States and the world. In many hospitals, the once clinical and impersonal settings called "labor and delivery" are being remodeled as homelike rooms. The philosophy of maternity care is being revolutionized.

"It's exciting!" exclaims the birthing-unit nurse manager of a hospital whose staff recently adopted a noninterventive approach to maternity care in which medical procedures are used only when needed. "I've been working here twenty years and for the first time, I think we're finally almost to the point where laboring women, I should say, families, are having babies the way they should."

A number of factors have contributed to the changes taking place in hospitals. One is the increasing popularity of home and childbearing-center birth. In California, a state where in some suburbs the rate of home births was 10 percent during the mid-1970s, the number of alternative-birth rooms in hospitals increased from three in 1975 to over 120 in 1982. This development of in-hospital birth alternatives is in part an attempt to mimic home birth. The women's movement, with its emphasis on women taking control of their own bodies and health care, has influenced many hospitals. In addition, consumer-oriented childbirth-education classes have made an increasing number of parents aware of their birth options and the disadvantages and risks involved in conventional obstetrics, medical interventions, and procedures. The resulting consumer pressure for a more humanized birth experience is inspiring hospitals to make changes. Finally, many childbirth professionals, particularly nurses—who are often the most instrumental in triggering change—are becoming increasingly aware of the psychological and emotional dimensions of labor. They are beginning to realize that peace, privacy, a positive emotional climate, and a supportive birth partner all work toward contributing to maternal–infant health.

HOW SAFE IS HOSPITAL BIRTH?

Most American parents and physicians take the safety of hospital birth for granted, assuming that the hospital is the safest birth environment. However, this is more of a sociocultural belief than a scientific fact. Many are surprised to hear that there is not a single medical study proving hospital birth to be safer than planned home or childbearing-center birth for the essentially normal mother.

Proponents of hospital birth point out that unforeseen complications are better handled in the hospital setting than elsewhere. Whether that makes the hospital safer or not, the majority of American mothers—including those interested in an alternative-birth experience—give birth in hospitals.

Though hospital birth *is* safe for most mothers, medical studies have shown that there is an increased risk of maternal and infant morbidity in the hospital as compared to home. The risk of infection to mother and baby is greater in the hospital (where there are more pathogenic organisms) than at home. In fact, the first U.S. rooming-in program, established in the 1940s at Duke University in North Carolina, was created not to promote maternal–infant attachment but to avoid severe nursery epidemics of infant diarrhea.

Varying with the hospital, the mother and baby are also at higher risk of iatrogenic complications. These include such problems as fetal distress from overuse of oxytocic drugs to stimulate labor and from pain-relief medication, infections from too many vaginal exams, and unnecessary surgical birth.

The postpartum baby blues is also significantly more common following hospital than home or childbearing-center birth. In a British study, pediatrician Aidan MacFarlane showed that 68 percent of hospital-birth mothers experienced baby blues compared to 16 percent of home-birth mothers.

Giving birth in a hospital with an emotionally positive climate where noninterventive obstetric care is the norm can dramatically reduce all these risks.

ADVANTAGES OF HOSPITAL BIRTH

The hospital is the safest environment for the mother at risk of medical complications during labor. Women with medical problems such as heart disease or diabetes or complications such as preeclampsia are best off in the hospital, where medical intervention is immediately available.

Emergency obstetric care is available if the mother develops complications at the last minute. An emergency cesarean delivery can be performed immediately.

*The mother avoids the rush of a last-minute transfer if medical prob-
lems develop and she must leave home or a childbearing center for
the hospital.* "If the home-birth mother develops problems and
must be transferred, moving from one end of town to the other by
ambulance is very inconvenient," says Richard Stewart, M.D., of
the Douglas Childbearing Center.

Many women feel safest and most comfortable in the hospital. Many
feel secure giving birth in a homelike setting in the hospital with the
knowledge that the latest technological equipment and expert care
are just a step away.

*Immediate pediatric attention is available should the baby have
medical problems.* Intensive care and a pediatrician or neonatolo-
gist are available twenty-four hours a day in most hospital facilities.
In some hospitals, however, a baby requiring intensive care often
must be transferred to another facility with an intensive-care center. (See page 176 for distinguishing care characteristics of
hospitals.)

DISADVANTAGES OF HOSPITAL BIRTH

Despite the benefits, hospital birth also carries a number of risks
and disadvantages. Many parents and professionals who have experienced both hospital and home birth feel that even the best hospital settings can't quite compare with the parents' own home. "Hospital birth—regardless of how beautiful the environment and how
supportive the staff—can never quite match home birth for peace
and comfort," says Dr. Howard Marchbanks, a physician who attends births in homes, childbearing centers, and hospitals in
Orange County, California.

And even the best hospitals don't have quite the positive emotional climate of childbearing centers. As Eunice Ernst of the National Association of Childbearing Centers puts it: "The hospital
alternative-birth setting is a quantum leap away from the free-
standing birth center. It is an attempt to accommodate the acute-
care setting to women who are not sick."

Disadvantages vary from one institution to another. There are
far fewer disadvantages in hospitals that have the qualities of a
good birth setting. Other disadvantages, as discussed in the opening chapters, include the following.

The risk of iatrogenic complications and infection to mother and baby is greater among mothers planning a hospital birth than among those planning a home or childbearing-center birth.

The mother is at a significantly higher risk of having an unnecessary cesarean section. This is more likely in a hospital with a high cesarean rate. Though some cesareans save the life of mother and/or baby, the vast majority are avoidable. It is far more difficult to avoid unnecessary surgery in a hospital with a 25- to 30-percent cesarean rate than it is in a childbearing center with only a 3- to 4-percent rate. (This rate refers to mothers transferred to the hospital for cesareans that are usually necessary. Again, childbearing centers screen for low-risk pregnancies, so of course their rate is lower.)

The father is often less actively involved in the childbearing process in the hospital than he is in the childbearing center or at home.

The parents are not on home ground. They do not have the same control as they do at home.

Hospitals are associated with illness. Birth is a normal, natural event, not an illness.

Most hospitals are not restful. Actually, some cite the ability to get rest as an advantage of hospital birth because they can remain in the hospital longer than in some birth centers if they prefer. But the quality of the rest they can get in a hospital is questionable. Few hospitals provide truly restful environments. As one nurse I know puts it: "If rest is your goal, it would be better to turn to the experts in the field; namely, the hotel and resort industry."

SETTINGS FOR ALTERNATIVE BIRTH IN THE HOSPITAL

A wide range of settings are available in today's hospitals for labor, birth, and the early postpartum period. Being acquainted with these will help you make the best choice among maternity hospitals in your area.

The Traditional Labor and Delivery Room

In traditional hospital birth, the mother labors in a labor room, usually a typical hospital room designed for one or two persons. Then, close to the time of giving birth, she is moved to a separate, sterile delivery room. After giving birth, she is moved to a third room called a recovery room. Then, anytime from minutes to hours afterward, she is moved to yet a fourth room on a postpartum unit. In conventional hospital delivery, the newborn is also typically transferred to no less than four rooms—from the delivery room to a transitional nursery, then to a newborn nursery, then to the mother's room for feeding (if the mother does not have twenty-four-hour rooming-in) and back again to the nursery.

Moving women and babies about from room to room during the childbearing process is one of America's most peculiar child-bearing customs. It is traumatic for the mother, who during labor is vulnerable and sensitive; upsetting for the father, who often must change into scrub clothes in a rush; a shock to the newborn; and a waste of hospital space and personnel hours. While a delivery room is a good setting for operative obstetrics because it is basically an operating room, it is about as suitable for beginning a family as a car wash is for celebrating a honeymoon.

This multitransfer form of obstetric care was modeled on the surgical system. Not long ago it was the rule in all maternity hospitals. Today, however, shifting childbearing women and babies around is rapidly becoming a procedure of the past as more and more health professionals realize that it serves no useful purpose and is a waste of time and money.

Alternative Facilities

Contemporary maternity facilities provide options where mother and baby can remain in the same room or, at most, two rooms throughout their hospital stay. These contemporary designs are re-placing the traditional labor and delivery-room setup and include the *birthing room,* the *labor-delivery-recovery room (LDR),* the *labor-delivery-recovery-postpartum room (LDRP),* and the *alternative birth center (ABC).*

When you think about it, there is really nothing new about the idea. Women have been laboring, giving birth, and remaining with their babies in the same room for as long as there have been homes. However, for hospitals, the idea was revolutionary and represented an entirely new concept in maternity care.

According to the American Hospital Association, as of 1987 nearly 80 percent of American hospitals had birthing rooms or other similar rooms (though not all of these hospitals use the single-room units regularly). The rooms vary as much as hotel rooms in appearance. Some are little different from ordinary labor rooms with a narrow bed and a nearby chair; others are beautifully furnished. Many have a single or double bed, pictures, wallpaper, comfortable chairs, and a private shower and/or bath.

Medical equipment and sterile instrument supplies are usually kept out of sight. For example, in the Family Birthing Center of Manchester Memorial Hospital, all medical equipment is kept in the hallways, close by but out of the parents' view. In a number of other birthing rooms I have visited, the medical supplies are kept in a closet that also contains an electronic fetal monitor and isolette for an infant requiring pediatric attention.

Some hospital settings, such as The Birth Place at St. Mary's Hospital in Minneapolis, have double beds. Unfortunately, however, most hospital maternity rooms have very narrow beds. This inhibits the mother from changing positions as she pleases and leaves little or no room for the father.

The lights can usually be dimmed as the parents desire. Most laboring women prefer a dimly lit room. The lighting should be subdued after the baby is born, as bright light hurts the sensitive newborn's eyes and will cause it to squint. In a dimly lit room, the infant will open its eyes and gaze at its parents' faces.

A traditional labor room can be used for both labor and birth if the parents wish and the hospital permits. This is the case in some hospitals that have not remodeled to create single-room maternity care. If birthing rooms, LDRs, or LDRPs are not yet available in your area, you may be able to arrange a labor-room birth in your local hospital with your caregiver's approval even if this is not standard hospital practice.

Birthing Rooms

In many states, the birthing room is defined as a room in a hospital providing family-centered care in a homelike environment for low-risk mothers throughout the labor, delivery, and immediate postpartum recovery period. However, some hospitals use the terms *birthing room*, *LDR*, and *LDRP* interchangeably.

The first birthing room in the United States was opened in 1969 at Manchester Memorial Hospital in Manchester, Connecticut, under the direction of pioneer obstetrician Dr. Philip Sumner. This hospital has recently remodeled and opened The Family Birthing Center, with six birthing rooms. All mothers give birth in these rooms, whether high- or low-risk. The only other rooms for birth are two "cesarean rooms," used solely for surgical delivery.

The care, policies, and atmosphere in birthing rooms vary tremendously from one institution to another. Some birthing rooms are tranquil, pleasant settings where noninterventive, individualized maternity care, flexible policies, and unrestricted contact with the baby after birth are the rule; others are characterized by highly interventive obstetric care and rigid policies.

In some hospitals, birthing rooms are little more than an advertising ploy. In one hospital where I assisted a woman through labor, there was no discernible difference in either policies or furnishings between birthing rooms and labor rooms.

When the mother and I arrived at the hospital, a nurse led us through a basement to what was called a "labor pod."

"What's a pod?" I asked.

"This is it," she said, indicating the entire labor and delivery area.

She then took us to a windowless, concrete cell with a narrow bed, a bed table with an electronic fetal monitor on top and a drawer stuffed with medical equipment, and a chair.

"Where are the birthing rooms?" I asked, still unsure what a pod was.

"These are the birthing rooms!"

It was a highly inappropriate environment to give birth. Throughout the mother's labor, loudspeakers blared constant interruptions, the nurses made us feel as welcome as a swarm of mosquitoes, and the policies were inflexible.

Don't depend on hospital literature for information on birthing rooms. Birthing rooms and other "alternative settings" frequently offer only the illusion of alternative birth. Sociologist Raymond DeVries, who has studied hospital birth alternatives, has pointed out that birthing rooms and similar settings within the hospital have imitated the physical environment of home while maintaining an interventive approach toward maternity care, medical control, and inflexible policies. In fact, his study of alternative-birth settings in the state of Washingon revealed no difference in labor options between hospitals with and without birthing rooms. Major obstetric interventions such as cesarean section and forceps delivery have actually increased in some hospitals with birthing rooms.

It is essential that you visit the birthing rooms and talk with the staff. For example, before making a final choice, Evelyn, a mother of two in central Vermont, visited several facilities. "The two larger hospitals in my area had birthing rooms," she recalls. "But the atmosphere was clinical and sterile. Policies unnecessarily restricted the mother's movements and the father's involvement. After talking with friends, we chose a small hospital with birthing rooms where laboring women were treated as people first, patients second."

WHEN YOU WON'T BE ABLE TO USE BIRTHING ROOMS

The requirements for using the birthing room vary widely from one hospital to another. In some states, regulations specify that birthing rooms are only for low-risk mothers. If medical problems such as fetal distress or elevated maternal temperature arise, the laboring woman must be transferred to a room more fully equipped for handling complications. A mother also may be transferred as a result of her request for medication, which is not available in many birthing rooms. If you want regional anesthesia such as an epidural, for example, the regulations of some states require that you be transferred to another room.

In some hospitals, rigid and often absurd requirements are placed on mothers who want to use the birthing room. For instance, some institutions' policies prevent many perfectly healthy women, such as those under or over a certain age or those planning a vaginal birth after a previous cesarean, from using the birthing room. Also, some hospitals require the mother and father to take special birthing-room classes before permitting them to use the alternative-birth setting.

Dr. Phillips warns parents to beware of hospitals that place these kinds of restrictions on alternative birth. Such restrictions indicate that the staff is not supportive of alternatives and may have a birthing room only as a marketing technique.

LDRs and LDRPs

Labor-Delivery-Recovery rooms (LDRs) and Labor-Delivery-Recovery-Postpartum rooms (LDRPs) are becoming the most popular option in maternity care. These units combine the homelike setting of the birthing room with the medical equipment and emergency support of a delivery room. While birthing rooms are generally limited to low-risk labors, LDRs accommodate both low- and high-risk labors. LDRs and LDRPs are also usually larger and more fully equipped than birthing rooms.

LDR rooms are designed for labor, birth, and the first hour or so after birth, after which the mother is moved to a postpartum unit. LDRP rooms are designed for the entire process of care for the mother through labor, birth, and the early postpartum period, as well as newborn care. Both rooms are fully equipped to handle most complications and obstetric procedures (except cesarean surgery). Both local and regional anesthesia can be used. The rooms are designed to accommodate the parents, guests the parents may invite, physician or midwife, pediatrician, anesthesiologist, scrub nurse, circulating nurse, obstetric resident, and students.

Many hospitals do not make a distinction between the terms *LDR* and *birthing room*. For example, St. Mary's Hospital in Grand Junction, Colorado has a maternity unit known as "The Family Birth Center." This consists of six rooms (called birthing rooms) where the mother labors, gives birth, and spends the first postpartum hour or so. She then has the option of being transferred to a mother–baby unit or going home. All mothers use these rooms regardless of risk status.

Hospitals with LDRs and LDRPs are beginning to or already have eliminated the use of the delivery room for anything but operative obstetrics. For example, at the Birthplace of St. Mary's Hospital in Minneapolis, Minnesota there are eighteen LDRP rooms, where the mother can remain from the moment she is admitted to the time she is discharged. Delivery rooms are used only for surgical birth, vaginal breech delivery, and multiple births.

CONDITIONS PREVENTING YOU FROM USING LDRs AND LDRPs

Requirements for using these rooms vary somewhat from one hospital to another. However, the most common conditions preventing the mother from using the LDR or LDRP or for transfer out of the unit include cesarean section, use of general anesthesia, presentations other than vertex, multiple births, and physician or client preference.

ADVANTAGES OF SINGLE-ROOM MATERNITY CARE

Utilizing the single-room LDRs or LDRPs has the following advantages over the multi-transfer system.

Increased safety. Emergencies requiring immediate medical attention can be handled more quickly, since there is usually no need to transfer the mother or newborn to another room. In addition, the risk of infection and injury during the move from one room to another is reduced.

A smoother, less traumatic labor. The laboring woman avoids the emotional trauma of moving from room to room, which can disrupt labor's progress.

Continuity of care. The mother usually has the same nurses for labor, delivery, and the early postpartum period. There are fewer unfamiliar faces and therefore fewer emotional adjustments to be made to the childbearing environment.

A more positive birth experience. Most parents greatly prefer remaining in a single homelike room throughout the childbearing process. When labor-delivery-recovery-postpartum suites were opened in one major Florida hospital, private-patient deliveries increased 126 percent. Other hospitals have noticed a similar increase in business after changing to a single-room care system.

Using a single room for labor, birth, and the postpartum period is less expensive than transferring clients from labor to delivery to recovery to postpartum room throughout the childbearing experience. In the multi-transfer system, more personnel is required. More linen must be changed and more rooms and equipment must be cleaned, increasing the cost of both supplies and staffing. The hospital and ultimately the consumer will save money as these options become more popular.

The Alternative Birth Center (ABC)

In some hospitals, an *alternative birth center* (ABC) is another word for a birthing room. In others, an ABC, also called a *family birth center* or *twenty-four-hour suite,* is a group of rooms for the family's use during the childbearing process. The ABC is actually a childbearing center within the hospital. For example, The Family Birthing Center owned by Providence Hospital in Southfield,

Michigan is a free-standing childbearing center consisting of very attractive single rooms where the family remains throughout labor.

The ABC represents what I consider the best option for hospital birth. ABCs may include a living room, small kitchen, and private bath in addition to a birthing room. The family uses this space from admission to discharge, which usually takes place within twenty-four hours after the baby is born. Medical equipment is kept out of sight but is readily available if needed.

Routine medical intervention, such as the use of IVs and electronic fetal monitoring, is less common in the ABC than in other hospital settings.

The Alternative Birthing Center of Hillcrest Medical Center in Tulsa, Oklahoma has a separate entrance so that parents do not have to feel as if they are entering a hospital with all the associations of illness. Each birthing suite consists of a private living room, family room, bathroom, and bedroom, as well as a kitchen families can share if they wish to prepare their own food. Parents can either bring their own food or order hospital food.

Unfortunately, ABCs like this are limited to a disappointingly small number of hospitals throughout the world. I hope that all maternity hospitals will one day provide this type of setting.

THE NURSING STAFF

The care the nurses provide, their attitudes, and their philosophy of childbirth can have a significant effect on your birth.

In the hospital, a nurse or nurses will probably be more actively involved during labor than your caregiver unless your caregiver is one who remains with mothers throughout labor (as do many midwives and even a few physicians). A nurse will check your baby's heart rate and your blood pressure, temperature, and pulse. In many hospitals, nurses also do vaginal exams to assess cervical dilation. (In some hospitals, a resident does this.)

Nursing care varies widely from hospital to hospital. In some institutions, a nurse remains with the mother throughout labor, providing one-to-one care; in others, nurses come and go to assess vital signs and labor's progress. Many mothers prefer to have a nurse present throughout labor, while others would rather be alone with their birth partner most of the time. If you want to be alone, simply tell the nurse that you and your partner would like privacy.

SETTINGS FOR ALTERNATIVE BIRTH IN THE HOSPITAL

The following can be comfortable settings conducive to a safe, positive labor, delivery, and early postpartum period. Bear in mind that setting alone does not create a rewarding birth. These settings are conducive to alternative birth only in hospitals with noninterventive maternity care, flexible policies, and supportive caregivers, as well as a nursing staff who view the mother as essentially healthy and accept the parents as the center of the childbearing drama.

Birthing room. A room where the mother labors, gives birth, and usually remains for the first postpartum hour or so. Birthing rooms are usually designed only for low-risk mothers. This term is sometimes used interchangeably with LDR, LDRP, and ABC.

Labor, delivery, recovery room (LDR). A room in which the mother (usually regardless of risk status) labors, gives birth, and spends the first hour or so after birth.

Labor, delivery, recovery, postpartum room (LDRP). A room in which the mother (usually regardless of risk status) labors, gives birth, and remains during the postpartum period throughout her hospital stay.

Alternative birth center (ABC), also called family birth center (FBC) or twenty-four-hour suite. A homelike facility for labor and birth consisting of a suite of rooms where the childbearing family remains from admission to discharge. In some hospitals, the term is used as a synonym for a birthing room, and it may also refer to a hospital-owned childbearing center.

In a few hospitals, nurses provide labor support in addition to health care. For example, at Bon Secours progressive maternity unit in Grosse Pointe, Michigan, all the nurses are skilled in helping the mother with breathing patterns, guided imagery, and other comfort measures, as well as in assisting the father to be involved in whatever way he wishes. Kathy Holland, R.N. and certified childbirth educator, says, "We are wholly committed to helping the mother and her partner achieve the kind of birth they want."

The Bon Secours nurses are eager to learn everything they can to better assist mothers through labor. As Kathy Holland points out: "We have discovered that guided imagery and deep relaxation is far more effective in helping the mother cope with labor than focusing primarily on the breathing patterns. So, we've all made the effort to learn this method."

In my experience conducting all-day workshops and observing nurses work with laboring mothers in hospitals throughout the United States, I have seen a surprising variation in nurses' outlooks on maternity care. In a few hospitals, the entire maternity nursing staff embraces the concepts characterizing alternative birth, including providing noninterventive obstetric care, viewing childbirth as a normal process, and respecting the parents' right to the kind of birth they want. In other institutions, nurses approach birth as a medical process and are unwilling or unable to meet the client's individual needs.

"I've found that some labor and delivery nurses have a tremendous amount of fear about birth," says Quila Rider, CNM of Orange County, California, who conducts training programs for registered nurses. "Many foreign-trained nurses have told me that the American system with its emphasis on technology and malpractice suits scares the Bejeebies out of them."

Meet the nurses when you visit the hospital to get an idea of their view of birth and the style of maternity care. If you plan to give birth in a hospital whose nursing staff does not share your views about childbirth, you can still achieve your goals, but you may have to work a little harder at reaching them. Here are some suggestions.

- Pay extra attention to labor support. Consider hiring a labor-support person to act as a consumer advocate.
- Provide the nursing staff with a copy of your birth plan signed by your caregiver.
- Meet with the head nurse or unit manager. Be specific and state precisely what you desire regarding your birth.
- Be polite but firm about your position if, during labor, a nurse insists on a particular procedure you wish to avoid.

Don't be intimidated if asked to sign a waiver of consent
form. This is required in many institutions if you refuse a
routine procedure.

PLANNING A HOSPITAL BIRTH

Having a safe, positive hospital birth with most of the benefits associated with alternative birth takes careful planning, including a
wise choice of institution. There are two major steps to take in
planning a rewarding hospital-birth experience: choosing a caregiver who supports your birth plans and choosing the best hospital
in your area.

In addition, you may want to consider hiring a childbirth assistant to help you achieve your personal plans and to provide additional emotional and physical support in the unfamiliar environment. A childbirth assistant can go a long way toward helping you
create an alternative birth in a hospital that is still learning about
this option or in a facility where alternative birth is not the norm.
Unfortunately, however, some hospitals don't permit such support
persons in addition to the father, so you should investigate the policy of any hospital you are considering.

Before she became a CNM, Quila Rider worked both as a registered nurse on a busy labor and delivery unit and, with another
woman, provided a childbirth-assistance service to women giving
birth in hospitals in her area. "My partner and I would both meet
with the woman first, so we could get to know her, and second, so
we could help her develop a birth plan," she says. "The birth plan
would include a statement of what she wanted in the birth. We
would help her negotiate over a period of weeks or months, if necessary, with the hospital nurses, particularly the nursing supervisor,
physicians, and sometimes even the perinatologist she might be visiting. We could get in writing a final birth plan signed by all appropriate persons. This was tremendously effective in helping parents
achieve their goals."

CHOOSING THE BEST HOSPITAL

"People often ask us why we traveled so far for our child's birth and
whether or not it was worth the inconvenience," says one mother
who carefully chose her maternity hospital. "Traveling twice the

distance would have been worth it. When you're in labor, you are hurt and scared. It is no time to fight for your rights. We were supported for our decisions rather than being made to feel as though our needs were inconveniencing anyone. We were encouraged in a natural and gentle birth the way we wanted it."

Some parents choose their caregiver first, then select the hospital. Others select the hospital, then look for a caregiver who practices there. In either case, it is worth spending the time and effort to select the best possible birth setting in your area. Following are some suggestions to make sure the hospital you choose is the best for you.

Visit the hospitals in your area and talk to the staff before making a final choice. Meet with some of the staff to find out whether they are committed to noninterventive obstetric care. This is of much greater importance than the physical setting. You can have a much more positive birth in a conventional delivery room with sensitive staff who individualize their care than you can in a birthing room with staff who view the mother as an ill patient and who adhere to rigid policies.

Formulate a verbal or written birth plan specifying your wishes regarding health-care options from labor to discharge. Hospitals vary dramatically in their routines and protocol. For example, even in birthing rooms, mothers and newborns are sometimes separated. However, you can request that your infant be examined, eye drops and the vitamin K shot be administered, and other newborn procedures take place while you or the father holds the newborn.

When you visit the hospital, ask questions to help you assess the birth place. Address your questions to nurses, the head nurse, or the unit manager. See page 180 for questions you may want to ask.

Find out the criteria for using the birthing room, LDR, LDRP, or ABC. In some hospitals, only so-called low-risk mothers are permitted to use these options. Overly strict screening requirements may exclude even perfectly normal women, such as those who are planning a vaginal birth after a previous cesarean. A few hospitals will require special birthing-room classes.

Find out about the criteria for transfer. Some hospitals have a high
rate of transferring mothers out of birthing rooms and alternative-
birth centers. Mothers are frequently moved to conventional labor
and delivery rooms for minor complications as well as for medical
emergencies. Also, in some hospitals women are not allowed to
have pain-relief medication or Pitocin-augmented or induced labors in the alternative settings. Therefore, if the mother feels she
needs pain relief, or if her caregiver opts to use Pitocin, she is moved
to a more conventional setting.

Be a shrewd consumer. Don't be misled by words and expressions
like "progressive" and "family-centered maternity care." Sometimes *progressive* refers only to the policy about raising hospital in-
come! The only way to know whether or not a hospital supports
alternative birth is by visiting the hospital, interviewing the staff,
and talking with parents who have given birth there.

Find out about admission procedures in advance of labor. Find out
what papers can be filled out in advance and complete them. Labor
is no time for *either* parent to have to answer a lot of questions and
fill out forms.

A GOOD HOSPITAL BIRTH

In the course of educating obstetrics professionals, I have had the
opportunity to participate in hundreds of births in scores of hospitals throughout the nation. These range from small hospitals with
less than two hundred births a year to huge teaching institutions
with ten thousand births yearly and include hospitals with rooms
ranging from simple and plain to those matching elegant hotel
suites. Regardless of the types of setting you consider, you should
look for *all* of the following characteristics when making your
choice.

A safe environment for birth. Make sure there is an anesthesiologist
available around the clock in case you need an emergency cesarean
section. There should be facilities to set up for surgery within no
more than thirty minutes. For the mother with medical complications, a safe hospital may mean an acute-care center. However,
most mothers are perfectly safe in a primary-care facility.

The quality of the medical care and maternal–infant safety should have top priority in your choice of hospital. However, a hospital-birth environment can be safe and still have all the additional qualities previously discussed.

TYPES OF HOSPITALS

When choosing a hospital it's important you know the three basic types of hospitals. These classifications are determined by the availability of emergency medical care.

A *level I facility, or primary-care center,* is a hospital that provides health care to low-risk clients. Its services include the identification of high-risk pregnancies, the provision of emergency care during unanticipated obstetric or newborn emergencies, and the care of normal newborns. Level I facilities are frequently in sparsely populated areas. Often there is no anesthesiologist in the birth unit, and it may take thirty minutes or more to set up for cesarean section.

A *level II facility, or secondary-care center,* is a hospital that offers care to the majority of clients and is able to provide care in about 90 percent of maternal or neonatal complications as well as low-risk care. Level II facilities are usually located in suburban areas. It usually takes only five to ten minutes to set up for an emergency cesarean in such a facility.

A *level III facility, or tertiary-care center,* is a hospital that provides care for high-risk clients who require the most sophisticated types of medical and technical intervention. Full-time specialists and the most modern equipment are available around the clock, and emergency cesareans can be done immediately. The tertiary-care center is best for certain life-threatening emergencies, neonatal surgery, very premature labors, and other medical complications. However, the atmosphere is usually highly clinical and therefore not ideal for normal birth.

Attractive and comfortable rooms. Attractively furnished rooms are obviously more appealing and relaxing than sterile cubicles or rooms painted in clinical green. However, a birth place need not be beautiful as long as it is comfortable for you. One of the best and safest family-centered hospitals I visited had simple, unadorned birthing rooms. Often the unintrusive health care and the staff's wholehearted commitment to serving your individual needs will more than make up for the lack of beautiful decor.

A staff who encourages you to determine the elements of your health care from admission to discharge. As one nurse put it: "This means giving the mother complete control to the degree that she wants to take it. If she wants to give birth standing up on the way back from the bathroom, that's what we help her do. We are here to support her choice providing it does not endanger her or her baby's health."

A staff who welcomes the father (or other birth partner) to remain with the mother throughout labor, birth, and the postpartum period regardless of where or how the phases of the childbearing process occur. The birth partner should be welcome to remain through all procedures, including preoperative preparation for cesarean birth, administration of anesthesia, cesarean surgery whether or not you are awake, and the entire postpartum period. Most hospitals welcome the father during vaginal birth. However, there are still some hospitals that deny him the right to witness the birth of his child if the mother has a cesarean, particularly if general anesthesia is used. "There is no excuse for this behavior," says prominent West Coast obstetrician Dr. Donald Creevy, Clinical Assistant Professor at Stanford University School of Medicine. "No health professional, regardless of his or her motive, should ever separate family members before, during, or after birth regardless of how the birth takes place."

A staff who views the father as an integral part of the family, never a visitor. An increasing number of hospitals are making this distinction: visitors should come and go during certain hours but fathers can remain with their family at any time, twenty-four hours a day if they desire.

Flexible policies the staff will bend to better serve the family's needs. Hospital policies vary widely. In some hospitals, policy is rigidly followed; in others, staff will bend policies to meet your needs.

For example, Chris Petrone, head of prenatal education at Manchester Memorial Hospital, says: "Individual flexibility underscores the basic philosophy of obstetrical care here. We recognize that families have individual needs and preferences and we try to accommodate them rather than expecting them to accommodate us. The mother can give birth in the position of her choice; the father can deliver the baby if he wants, or he can cut the cord; children can attend births, surrogate parents can attend—whatever the parents want."

The freedom for the mother to invite the guests of her choice (family, friends, her children, labor-support persons) to share her labor and birth. A hospital that denies the mother the guests of her choice is not giving her preference top priority. The common excuse that there is no room or that guests will interfere with others' privacy is often invalid. Most hospitals that deny a mother the company she wishes still find room to accommodate medical and nursing students.

Freedom to walk around as the mother pleases during labor. In a hospital that encourages natural birth, the mother is free to move about unless there is a medical complication requiring bed rest. For many women, walking and remaining upright during labor hastens its progress and reduces discomfort.

Freedom to shower, take baths, or use a Jacuzzi as the mother wishes. An increasing number of hospitals have bathtubs or Jacuzzis for laboring women. During active labor warm water can relax the mother, reduce pain, and in many cases hasten labor's progress, yet many hospitals restrict mothers with ruptured membranes from taking tub baths. This policy is designed to lower the risk of infection, which increases once the membranes have ruptured. However, if you are in active labor, there is not enough time for an infection to develop.

No routine medical procedures for the essentially healthy laboring woman. Such procedures as shaving of the perineal area, administration of an enema, intravenous feeding, continuous or intermittent electronic fetal monitoring, artificial rupture of the fetal membranes, and cutting an episiotomy should not be done unnecessarily.

Encouragement of breastfeeding. This means the mother who plans to breastfeed receives support to breastfeed exclusively. *No* routine bottles of formula or water are given to the baby.

No separation of healthy infants and mothers at any time throughout the hospital stay. Many hospitals that advertise rooming-in often place infants in the nursery at certain times, such as during visiting hours.

Privileges granted to certified nurse-midwives as well as physicians. Any hospital with your needs at heart will willingly grant privileges to CNMs. This does not necessarily mean there are midwives on staff, as there may simply be no midwives practicing in the area. The important factor is that the hospital has an open door to midwives.

Family-centered maternity care. This is a philosophy of care that focuses on the psychological and social needs of the mother, father, newborn, and other family members, as well as the mother's physical needs. In a hospital that embraces true FCMC, the mother's obstetric care is individualized to meet her personal needs; fathers are welcome to be involved throughout the entire labor and birth process regardless of whether the baby is born vaginally or via cesarean section; labor and birth take place in a homelike setting; no restrictions are placed on children participating during labor and birth, visiting their mothers, and interacting with their newly born sibling; and the hospital has a program of early discharge so the mother can adapt to the first few days of new parenthood in her own home.

Though a valid and important concept, FCMC can be a misleading term. For example, some hospitals claiming to be family-centered prohibit children from visiting the first hours after birth, and a few will not permit fathers to attend cesareans, particularly if general anesthesia is used.

"Be wary of such places," warns Dr. Celeste Phillips, R.N. Ed.D. "Hospitals that separate family for *any* reason are not good places for childbearing."

In their book *Family Centered Maternity Care,* Professor Susan McKay and Dr. Celeste Phillips point out: "Comprehensive FCMC is not well-decorated birthing rooms with flowered wallpaper, . . . nor is it birthing chairs or birthing beds . . . restrictive policies and protocols often dominate care. In such settings, parents are 'allowed' to hold their baby, and siblings are 'permitted' to touch their new brother or sister only with physicians' orders and only during certain time periods. Such restrictions make it very obvious to the family just who is in charge, i.e., the professional staff."

Acceptance of home-birth midwives and physicians should a mother plan to give birth at home and have to be transferred to a hospital at the last minute. Even if you are not planning a home birth, asking the staff about their reactions to women planning to give birth at home can help you evaluate their attitude toward meeting your needs.

QUESTIONS TO ASK THE HOSPITAL

The answers to the following questions can help you assess whether or not a hospital supports alternative birth and is the right place for you and your baby. You can direct these questions to staff nurses, the head nurse on the birthing unit, or an administrator.

- Is nursing care provided on a one-to-one basis? If not, how many laboring women does each nurse care for?
- Are any medical procedures (intravenous feeding, continuous electronic fetal monitoring, and so forth) routine? If continuous electronic fetal monitoring is not routine, is monitoring routine at any time during labor?
- If any procedures are routine, what percentage of mothers ask to have them waived?
- How does the staff react when a mother or father asks that a routine procedure be waived?
- Do laboring women have a private bathroom? Shower? Bath?
- Is the mother free to shower or bathe during labor? Can she use the bathtub or Jacuzzi whether or not her membranes are ruptured?
- Is the mother encouraged to eat lightly and drink liquids as she wishes during labor?
- Is the mother free to walk around as she pleases throughout labor?
- Can women give birth in the position of their choice?

- Are stirrups commonly used for delivery?
- What percentage of mothers use the birthing room?
- Are there any restrictions on using the birthing room? If so, what are they?
- What percentage of women are transferred out of the birthing room? What are the most common reasons for transfer? (Look for a lower percentage of transfers than 5 to 6 percent.)
- Are fathers (or other birth partners) welcome to remain with the mother throughout all procedures, including pre-operative administration of anesthesia, cesarean surgery, and postoperative recovery?
- May the mother invite whomever she wishes, including children, to share her labor and birth?
- Do certified nurse-midwives have privileges?
- What is the cesarean rate?
- Are mothers encouraged to breastfeed? Do breastfed babies routinely receive bottles of water or formula?
- Are healthy infants and mothers separated for any reason? (At night? During visiting hours?)
- How many mothers choose to go home within two to six hours after giving birth?
- Are children welcome to see and hold the healthy newborn within the first hour after birth?
- Can fathers room with the mother and baby twenty-four hours a day?

If You Are a High-Risk Mother

Pregnancy or labor is considered high-risk if there are previous medical, current obstetric, or socio-economic conditions that are potentially dangerous to the health and/or life of the mother or baby. The mother with a potentially complicated labor requires more watchful medical care and, in many cases, medical intervention. The increased likelihood of special needs limits her options. For example, the mother who would benefit from intravenous medication or continuous electronic fetal monitoring may have less mobility and may not be able to give birth in the position of her choice.

However, all mothers—regardless of risk status—will benefit from giving birth in an emotionally positive climate where their psychological as well as physical needs are met. For that matter, the mother at high risk may benefit even more from the qualities associated with alternative birth than the essentially healthy mother. During labor, such a mother often experiences feelings of failure, guilt, and anxiety. Being in a comfortable birth setting, surrounded by family and supportive loved ones, can help her and her mate experience a positive birth even in the presence of complications.

In a few hospitals, the high-risk mother has these options. For example, at the University of Utah Medical Center in Salt Lake City, mothers with medical complications are welcome to use the birthing rooms. In fact, a special birthing room for high-risk mothers adjoins a nursery.

The mother and baby with medical problems can benefit by eliminating the last-minute rush to the delivery room. As Richard B. Stewart, M.D., says: "We don't transfer clients from one room to another if complications arise or the mother requests medication. If complications develop, the family remains with the mother."

However, in the majority of hospitals, only women who are expected to have perfectly normal deliveries are candidates for an alternative-style birth. As Susan McKay and Celeste Phillips point out, "Segregation of families so that some are eligible for family-centered intrapartum [labor] care while others are not is discriminatory and masks the goal of a family-centered program—that is, to provide for the needs of all family members, regardless of the specifics of the birth experience."

With proper preparation, the siblings of a high-risk infant can benefit from being included during labor or in the immediate postpartum period. They should be welcomed to visit the sick newborn in the intensive-care unit. This will enhance siblings' acceptance of the infant and will have a positive effect on the entire family.

In some hospitals, however, siblings are prevented from visiting the sick infant. This policy is based on the notion that the presence of family will increase the risk of infection. However, hospitals already have far more pathogenic infection-causing microbes than anyone is likely to bring in from outside, and family members are just as capable of scrubbing their hands as medical professionals. In fact, one study conducted by pioneer pediatrician John Kennel showed that the family members were even more careful about hand-washing!

Even if you can't change them, being aware of these policies will help your birth experience to go smoother.

If You Can't Find an Ideal Hospital Near Your Home

If you have the choice, of course it is preferable to select a hospital where alternative birth is the norm. Unfortunately, in some areas there are no hospitals that support alternative birth. If this is the case in your area, you may still be able to plan the birth you want.

Many hospitals that do not yet encourage the kind of birth experience described in this book are ripe for change. For example, I am often invited to conduct workshops in hospitals whose nursing staff appear to be quite conventional. However, the nurses often turn out to be eager to learn new ways to support the mother through labor, get the father involved in the childbearing process, and see hospital policies changed.

In one hospital where I was to lecture, birthing rooms had replaced the combination labor-and-delivery-room setup. However, women remained in bed during active labor. The nurse manager of the laboring and delivery unit asked me to tell parents that it was okay to get out of bed during labor. "But I thought it was hospital policy . . . ," I started to say, when she interrupted me. "That's why I can't tell them!" she said. "The doctors don't want to change. The only ones who can change this place are the parents and the nurses!"

You may be able to plan the birth you want simply by asking for it. In fact, the obstetric staff in some hospitals may welcome your request. However, it's best not to depend on this: some hospitals will refuse to deviate from policy.

To maximize your chance of a positive birth experience in a less-than-ideal situation, take the following steps.

- Choose a caregiver who is as supportive as possible of your goals.
- Draw up a written birth plan. Discuss your plan with the staff and be prepared to make compromises.
- Consider hiring an experienced childbirth assistant to interface with staff and see that your birth plans are followed.
- Consider temporarily relocating to be near a hospital that offers alternative-birth options. Many parents travel to friends' or relatives' homes in other cities.

RESISTANCE TO ALTERNATIVE BIRTH
WITHIN THE HOSPITAL

Creating the setting for an alternative birth within the hospital is a long-term process. It means changing the attitudes of caregivers and nurses. For example, when the Birthplace at St. Mary's Hospital in Minneapolis was opened, many nurses had to develop a new view of the childbearing family. "The change was slow and painful," recalls head nurse Colleen Gerlach. A full third of the staff, who were unable to accept the change, left.

When Dr. Richard Stewart conceived of the Douglas Birthing Center in Douglasville, Georgia, he at first faced tremendous resistance to his ideas. The main issue physicians most opposed was Dr. Stewart's plan for midwives to do deliveries without a physician present. "Normal healthy women with uncomplicated pregnancies need midwives, not doctors," he insisted.

Physicians also resisted Dr. Stewart's practice of discharging mother and baby within six to eight hours after birth. Now most health practitioners realize that early discharge enables mothers to make a smoother transition to parenthood. However, discharge within twenty-four to forty-eight hours is still the rule in many hospitals and childbearing centers across the nation.

Like the opposition to midwives and the prejudice against home birth, resistance to hospital-birth alternatives is not entirely based on reason. Several factors contribute to the resistance.

Some physicians and nurses find it hard to accept the parent-directed obstetric care and the lack of established routine that characterize alternative birth. They are uncomfortable with the father's active role during labor, the mother's family and perhaps friends being allowed to come and go, and the mother being able to walk around as she pleases and to give birth in the position of her choice.

Many childbirth professionals resist losing control of the childbearing process. As Colleen Gerlach recalls, "Making the change meant a lot of letting go on the part of the nurses. They had to learn to give up control and allow the childbearing family to make decisions. In the old system, we made all the decisions. We managed the labor. Now, in the new system, we support the family."

Alternative birth requires viewing childbirth in an entirely different way than most physicians and nurses have been taught. The practitioner must be reeducated about childbirth and learn to view the mother as a healthy client rather than an ill patient. This takes time and a healthy dose of patience.

Some find the flexible policies difficult to accept and to put into action. They are used to one-size-fits-all obstetric care and have difficulty meeting the needs of individuals with a variety of birth plans.

Nurses with training and experience in obstetric technology sometimes find it difficult to work in a less intervention-oriented environment. The head nurse of one busy unit told me, "We used to believe that electronic fetal monitoring was beneficial with all patients regardless of risk status. The studies showed that EFM could actually be hazardous with low-risk women. Conscientious practitioners discontinued routine EFM. Then we believed it could help the high-risk, was mandatory for the high-risk. Now the studies show that EFM may be hazardous with high-risk. But the staff continues using the machine!"

Some physicians find the alternative-birth setting less convenient for them. They prefer standing at the delivery table to stooping over a low bed to "catch" a baby.

With experience, most health professionals learn to adapt to the philosophy and setting associated with alternative birth. After having participated in a number of deliveries, they discover that alternative birth is not only safe, but a more positive experience for the entire family and therefore more satisfying for the practitioner.

Susan Driesel, the head of the women's health center at Hillcrest Medical Center in Tulsa, Oklahoma, has seen a dramatic change take place in the attitudes of her staff: "Many physicians and nurses felt that alternative birth was unsafe, risky, and that there would never be a demand for it. It just didn't fit in with their paradigm. It didn't have a place in what they considered acceptable practice. When Hillcrest opened the Alternate Birth Center, physicians and nurses who were skeptical of alternative birth had the opportunity to witness the support mothers received. This gradually dispelled their fears. They could see alternatives such as freedom of mobility, the presence of support persons of the mother's choice, laboring without intravenous feeding or monitoring, working in that environment. They learned to accept these things and incorporate them into the traditional environment."

LOOKING AHEAD

A statement published by the New York Academy of Medicine concludes: "Efforts should be made to establish a more widely effective home-like family centered birthing environment within the hospital setting."

The alternative-birth setting is still an evolving concept. Hospitals are still learning how to create an environment most conducive to normal labor and a positive beginning to the life-long adventure of parenthood, and health professionals are still learning to adapt philosophy and setting to match that of home birth. We have a long way to go, and the hospital will probably never be quite like home.

However, out-of-home birth continues to improve. Perhaps the day is not far off when every maternity hospital will have birthing suites like the hospitals discussed in this chapter. And gradually, the health-care providers who take part in the dramatic adventure of giving birth may adopt the philosophy that makes alternative birth so different from conventional hospital obstetrics.

One nurse manager summed it up: "It takes courage to change, to let go of old habits, sometimes to completely rethink what you have been taught, and to see the mother as a client who has the right to dictate to us what she wants (even if we don't agree). A lot of nurses just aren't willing to make that change. For them, there are other hospitals. But for those who choose to remain here and ride the change out, there is no turning back. You cannot experience alternative birth and ever want it any other way."

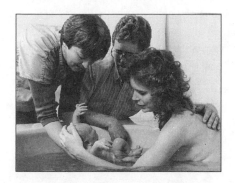

CHAPTER 8

Waterbirth

ANNE RIVERS'S FIRST CHILD was born in a military hospital. After giving birth, Anne and her newborn were separated for twelve hours. For the next three days she saw her baby only once every four hours for bottle feedings. It was a frightening and painful experience for her.

Her second child was born twelve years later in a mountain home in Oregon. When she was pregnant with her third child, Anne planned for the birth to take place at home, but as a result of complications she had to transfer to a hospital. The staff was overbearing. Once again she felt totally powerless in a hospital environment.

"I wanted to create the most positive and supportive birth possible for my fourth child," Anne recalls. She had read about experienced waterbirth midwives in Hawaii. Excited about the possibility of having a waterbirth herself, she and her family packed their bags and moved to Maui. They were able to find a house and a midwife fairly quickly, and Anne began making her birth arrangements six weeks before her due date.

Once in active labor, Anne slipped into the tub. Near the time of birth, her husband and two of her other children also got into the tub. The baby was born into the warm water. Anne says, "My two-year-old stood next to me on the low seat and was the first to speak: 'That's my baby.'"

Noelani rested a minute underwater before Anne gently lifted her to the surface, bringing her to her breast. "A few sputters, a muffled whimper, and she was breathing," she says. "I slid her back into the warm water. She was content to lie back, accustomed to the weightlessness and warmth of the water. I cradled the back of her little head in my palm. She floated, arms outstretched, eyes wide, calmly taking in her new home. We sat together, a bond of warm water flowing around and between us."

Anne's six-year-old son had stayed with her throughout the labor. After the birth, he patted her on the back and said: "That was a great birth, Mom!"

Anne still lives in Maui. Today she is a midwife helping other families discover the beauty of waterbirth.

WHAT IS WATERBIRTH?

"The affinity of pregnant women for water is still a mystery to us," says Dr. Michel Odent. "Many mothers-to-be say that they are drawn to water; they feel a strong urge to dive into the waves, or dream of floating on the surface for long periods of time. Some women who are strongly drawn to water throughout pregnancy are even more attracted to it during labor. Still others tell us that they don't like the water or can't swim. Yet as labor begins, these same women will suddenly move toward the pool, enter eagerly, and not want to leave!"

An innovative and controversial alternative, waterbirth was first popularized in the 1960s in the Soviet Union by Russian researcher Igor Charkovsky. A unique and brilliant scientist, Dr. Charkovsky has been called the "father of waterbirth." He uses rectangular Plexiglas tanks six feet long, two feet wide, and two-and-a-half to three feet deep for the birth. The mother can move into whatever position is most comfortable for her. She can use both sides of the tank for support, someone else can get in the tank with her, and persons assisting at the birth can easily reach inside. The Plexiglas also allows whoever is attending the birth to clearly see what is going on.

French physician Dr. Michel Odent popularized waterbirth in Europe in the unique, wonderful, and now internationally famous maternity unit of a small hospital in Pithiviers, a town about an hour's drive from Paris.

In 1977, Dr. Odent made the warm-water pool available to laboring women to relieve pain, promote relaxation, and reduce the need for medication. At that time, he had not planned for women to give birth in the water. However, some laboring women felt so relaxed in the pool that, when it came time to give birth, they didn't want to leave. Taking his cue from the laboring women, Dr. Odent assisted them with waterbirth.

The birthing room in Pithiviers is designed to relax the mother and help her achieve the ideal state of mind for the optimal birth. Painted in earth tones, it includes a low, cushioned platform where the mother and others, who assist her or share the birth with her, can move freely. If the laboring woman wants, she can go to an adjacent room where there is a custom-made circular sky-blue pool, seven feet in diameter and two-and-a-half feet deep. The mother has plenty of room to immerse herself and change positions as she desires, and two people can move around freely.

In the years following Dr. Odent's *discovery,* most women at Pithiviers gave birth in the supported semisquatting position in the birthing room. However, many others chose to have waterbirths in the sky-blue circular pool. Most mothers are in a vertical position, kneeling in the water for the first moment of mother–infant contact. Dr. Odent told me that he doesn't emphasize waterbirth, but he feels it should be an option available to all laboring women.

So does California midwife Susanna Napierala. She has attended fifty waterbirths in places throughout the world, including California, Hawaii, the Caribbean, and the Soviet Union. She attended her first waterbirth in 1982 after learning about underwater delivery one evening while teaching childbirth classes.

"A couple asked if we could watch something on TV instead of having class," she recalls. Excerpts from a Swedish-made film called *Waterbabies* about Charkovsky's work with water-training and waterbirth was scheduled on a popular TV show. "I was indignant that they would rather watch TV than have class!" she says, laughing. "But we watched TV."

After watching a woman giving birth in the water, Rennie, a woman in the class, exclaimed, "That's for me!"

Susanna recalls: "I've always been a midwife who wanted to respect the needs of women giving birth. I've always felt that if a woman has her needs satisfied, she's going to give birth well."

She began to research waterbirth. Meanwhile, Rennie and her husband, Larry, made preparations to give birth in the water. Larry, who was an architect with experience in shipbuilding, built a water tank equipped with waterbed heaters to keep the water warm.

"Rennie was tense during labor, having a hard time," says

Susanna. "But once she got in the water, it was like watching a different person! She relaxed and let nature take its course. Rennie, Larry, someone else supporting Rennie, and I were in the tank. Rennie gave birth in a squatting position supporting herself on the ledge of the tank.

"I'll never forget when the head was born underwater. I thought: 'My God, what am I doing?' Then I reminded myself that it was perfectly safe. Everything was going to be okay.

"And it was. I'd attended about 300 births by that time, but this was the most beautiful birth I'd ever seen. When the baby was halfway out of her mother, she opened her eyes underwater and looked up at her father, then closed her eyes again. Somebody in the room whispered, 'She looks as if she is at perfect peace.' Another contraction came and Rennie pushed her daughter out. The baby was so peaceful she didn't even know she was born!

"When I saw how beautiful waterbirth could be, I began to help other women birth in the water."

At a conference of childbirth and other health professionals in Toronto sponsored by the Pre- and Perinatal Psychology Association of North America, Binnie Dansby, a midwife, called waterbirth "the ultimate alternative available in birthing practices at this time." She continued: "Emotionally and spiritually, waterbirth is a peaceful and gentle entry for the human being and its mother. Allowed to labor in water, the mother has a maximum amount of comfort and the choice of her bed or the water for the birth. The atmosphere is safe, secure, and warm. The laboring woman is supported by familiar people whom she has chosen and who are ready and willing to do whatever she wishes. There is the opportunity for the father to participate as fully as he chooses; couples report a deeper bond in their relationship, and fathers enjoy an immediate close relationship with the new baby."

Another couple, Dawn and Mike of Kent, England, were keen scuba divers for whom waterbirth seemed an appropriate option. They talked to their midwife, Linda Ford at Maidstone Hospital, one of those rare hospitals that favors total flexibility in the care of laboring women. Linda recalls, "I had no previous experience of underwater delivery, but promised to obtain as much relevant information as possible."

Mike made a water tank of his own and brought it into the hospital. When his and Dawn's daughter Jasmine was born underwater, "we all gazed at this most amazing sight," Linda remembers. "Just as we had been told, the baby made no attempt to open its eyes or to breathe. I was reminded of the pictures of the fetus in utero."

There was one complication which struck the new father with horror. Just after the birth, he realized he had not loaded his camera!

Convinced of the benefits of waterbirth, pioneer obstetrician Dr. Michael Rosenthal assists mothers with waterbirth at his child-bearing center in Upland, California. More waterbirths have occurred there, at The Family Birthing Center, than anywhere else in the United States. In March 1990, the center celebrated its six-hundredth waterbirth of the nearly two thousand births that have taken place there since it opened in 1985. Because The Family Birthing Center is one of the only American centers where water-birth is an available option, women travel from as far as Alaska and Montreal to give birth there. Two warm-water baths measuring six feet long, four feet wide, and eighteen inches deep are available for laboring women.

Other childbearing centers throughout the world are begin-ning to include waterbirth. For example, the Natural Childbirth In-stitute and Women's Health Center in Culver City, California has had about a dozen waterbirths over the past few months. The mid-wives plan to see more women use their newly installed tub for un-derwater delivery. Nearly three hundred babies have been born in the water at St. James Natural Childbirth Clinic in Malta, and al-most a hundred waterbirths have occurred in Federal Hospital in Obenpullendorf, Austria. Other hospitals such as the previously noted Maidstone in Kent are just beginning to learn about water-birth but are coming to accept it as a safe alternative.

Waterbirth is attracting an increasing number of parents, and advocates for this childbirth option are increasing yearly. An or-ganization called Waterbirth International (WBI) was founded by Barbara Harper, R.N., in Santa Barbara, California in 1989 to pro-vide information, referrals, videotapes, tub rentals, seminars, con-sultations, and prenatal classes for parents and professionals inter-ested in waterbirth. WBI's goal is, as Barbara puts it, "To turn the tide on the current high-tech, hospital, medically controlled ap-proach to childbirth back to family-centered birth where the intui-tion of the birthing woman is respected and the baby is included as a conscious participant in its own birth."

Barbara's own interest in waterbirth was triggered during the years following her hospital birth in 1978. "As a nurse who had worked OB and had taken Lamaze classes, I felt quite well-prepared for birth," she recalls. "But my experience was one of being robbed of what childbirth should have been—a beautiful, positive experience. I spent twenty-four hours lying on what the hospital called an alternative birthing-room bed, which was really little more than a delivery table with wheels. Since my labor was not progressing, I was given Pitocin to augment contractions. This made my contractions far more painful. Afterwards, I was extremely upset even though I gave birth to a beautiful daughter.

"Six years later when I was pregnant again, I began looking into alternatives. One midwife I interviewed had just returned from Pithiviers where, she told me, some babies were born in the water and birth was a peaceful and natural process without unnecessary medical intervention. At that time I could find no information on waterbirth, so I left Santa Barbara and flew to visit Michel Odent in France. While in Pithiviers, I attended a birth. I watched a young woman climb out of the pool where she had been laboring for some time and squat, supported by her husband, close to the floor where a white sheet had been spread. The midwife, Dominique, sat in front of her in complete silence. I was allowed into the birthing room only after I was instructed that it would be dark and completely silent. The only sounds were those beautiful primal sounds emanating from the birthing mother.

"Observing that beautiful birth changed my entire perspective of childbirth. My own second baby was born in 1984 in a home-constructed tub at the foot of my bed and my third was born in 1986 in our outdoor Jacuzzi."

Over the next few years, over a hundred women asked Barbara for information about waterbirth. She attended eight waterbirths, and five mothers came to her home to use her Jacuzzi for their births. To fill the need for educating parents and professionals about this gentle childbirth option, she founded Waterbirth International. Their address is located in the Resources at the end of this book.

As Dr. Rosenthal puts it: "There is nothing new about water. People have been using it for pain relief for thousands of years. It makes sense to use warm water for birth."

HOW SAFE IS WATERBIRTH?

Speaking of waterbirth at Pithiviers, Dr. Odent says, "We have found no risk attached either to labor or to birth underwater."

After his experience with over six hundred waterbirths at The Family Birthing Center, Dr. Rosenthal says he also has seen no complications.

The two problems parents and professionals are most concerned about are the mother developing an infection and the infant inhaling water with a possible risk of pneumonia or drowning.

Regarding the first concern, there is very little risk of infection to the mother providing the water is clean. Many health professionals advise expectant mothers to avoid tub baths once membranes have ruptured. When the amniotic sac has broken, there is a risk that bacteria may enter the uterus and cause infection. However, avoiding immersion in water is not necessary once the mother is in active labor, since there is no time for an infection to develop. "When labor is in progress," Dr. Rosenthal points out, "everything is headed downstream, inhibiting the passage of bacteria up the birth canal into the uterus even if there were time to develop an infection." Dr. Igor Charkovsky adds: "There is no risk involved in the husband being in the water with his wife either, since they share the same bacterial flora."

Waterbirth advocates agree that there is virtually no danger of the newborn drowning *if the baby is taken to the surface immediately after birth.* Dr. Odent says, "To this day, we have never needed to clear breathing passages after such a birth." He adds, "Women seem to know that it is not at all dangerous to give birth in water; there is no risk to the newborn, who, after all, has known only watery environments."

For a short while, the infant continues to "breathe" through the umbilical cord. The baby usually does not actually begin breathing on his or her own until reaching the air. Since water has been the baby's natural environment for nine months in the uterus, the newborn will not attempt breathing while submerged. Even if the baby were to gasp underwater, Dr. Charkovsky explains, an automatic reflex would shut off the windpipe as soon as water entered the throat. "We are not confronting the child with anything new," he asserts. "We are simply prolonging the conditions so beneficial to development. Living in the water is totally natural for a newborn. He's never done anything else."

Most waterbirth advocates agree that the safest approach is to bring the baby to the surface within no more than a minute or two after birth. Keeping the baby submerged is not advised. Even though the risk of drowning is slight, there is a risk that the baby can develop hypoxia (a condition of inadequate oxygen), which can cause brain damage. As Dr. Rosenthal points out: "Within seconds after the birth, the placenta begins to separate from the uterine wall because the amount of uterine wall surface has been enormously reduced and the placenta is not elastic enough to remain attached . . . the oxygenation of the fetal blood that is being brought to the placenta decreases immediately."

In her article in the *Journal of Nurse-Midwifery,* Linda Church, a midwife from The Family Birthing Center, adds: "Although the infant goes from one watery environment to another and does not take its first breath until its skin thermoreceptors are stimulated by air contact, it has minimal oxygen reserves. Because the placenta ceases to function as completely as before—even with a pulsating cord—once born, the infant is on its own and must be immediately lifted to the air to breathe."

Most waterbirth practitioners advise the mother to leave the tank before delivering the placenta. If the mother were to remain in the water at this time, Dr. Odent believes, she might be at a slight risk of developing a water embolism. That is, when the placenta detaches, a bubble of water could get into the mother's bloodstream and perhaps go to the head and cause a stroke. However, this is a theoretical risk; the event actually has never occurred.

At this time, there is little *documented* information about the safety of birth in the water. However, judging from the experience of responsible midwives and physicians who have participated in subaquatic delivery, it is assumed that waterbirth under the correct supervision is safe. As Dr. Rosenthal puts it: "The use of water for labor and birth is a sane, intelligent, practical, and safe procedure. It's humane, it restores control of birthing to women, and it eliminates the need for many medical interventions that are clearly counterproductive when compared to the amazingly simple intervention of allowing a woman to sit in warm water."

USING WATER IN THE CHILDBEARING PROCESS

While the term *waterbirth* is often used to refer to actually giving birth in the water, warm water can be used during childbearing in other ways, including labor in the water and the newborn bath.

Labor in the Water

Many women find it soothing to sit in a tub of warm water during active labor. For this reason, an increasing number of hospitals and birthing centers now include bathtubs, hot tubs, Jacuzzis, or whirlpools on the maternity unit. The mother usually labors in the tub, then gets out sometime before it is time to give birth.

Cindy, a mother from Indiana, recalls: "I'm not usually one for long baths but I must have spent half my labor in the bathtub! Nothing seemed to soothe me like the hot bath. My husband, Gary, spent most of the time pouring water over my abdomen and wondering when I'd be out of the tub."

Unfortunately, some hospitals equipped with Jacuzzis don't promote their use in pregnancy. Once, after lecturing at a hospital where a Jacuzzi had recently been installed, I asked a nurse whether she thought it was helpful to laboring mothers. "Women hardly ever get to use it," she said with obvious vexation about her hospital's policies.

Also, in many hospitals mothers are not allowed to use the Jacuzzi once membranes have ruptured. The Jacuzzi is used only during early labor, which is unfortunate, since it is during late active labor that the mother will most benefit from immersion in warm water.

A hot tub bath with the water as deep as possible can be particularly relaxing when contractions mount in intensity during late first-stage labor. Warm water also relieves the pain of labor contractions. In addition, immersion in a hot bath can facilitate labor's progress, helping the mother have a more efficient labor.

Researchers at the University of Copenhagen compared a group of laboring women who bathed in a hot tub bath for one-half to one hour with another group of laboring women who did not use the tub. They found the laboring women who spent time in the bath experienced pain relief as well as more rapid cervical dilation (2.5 centimeters per hour, as compared to 1.26 centimeters per hour in the nonbathing group).

Dr. Odent recommends waiting until the cervix has dilated five centimeters before getting in the warm water. He found that the warm-water bath can inhibit labor before five centimeters but enhance labor's progress after this point. However, most practitioners agree that the mother should enter the tub *whenever she wishes.*

Water may assist the mother to labor more efficiently in a number of ways. In an article for the prestigious British medical journal *The Lancet,* Dr. Odent says: "We believe that the warm pool facilitates the first stage of labor because of the reduction of the secretion of noradrenaline and other catecholamines [stress hormones]; the reduction of sensory stimulation when the ears are underwater; the reduction of the effects of gravity; the alteration of nervous conduction; the direct muscular stretching action; and peripheral vascular action."

There are other benefits of laboring in the water that are less easily analyzed. As Dr. Odent points out: "We have observed that water seems to help many parturients [mothers] reach a certain state of consciousness where they become indifferent to what is going on around them." He has also observed that sometimes just the sound of water rushing into the tub is enough to cause some women to progress from first- to second-stage labor. In addition, some caregivers have observed that laboring in the water lowers the mother's inhibitions. Decreased inhibitions may allow the woman to surrender to labor more readily and thereby labor more efficiently.

Dawn, the mother who gave birth in a tank of warm water in Maidstone Hospital, recalls: "The tank was still being filled and the water was not at the required depth. Nevertheless, all I wanted to do was strip off and jump in and that is exactly what I did."

A hot shower can also be relaxing. The mother can stand under the shower and let the water play over her back and abdomen. One laboring woman used the shower for the dual purpose of relaxing and avoiding a nurse who was attempting to hook her up to an electronic fetal monitor. Since the baby's heart tones had proved healthy, the mother saw no reason to use the monitor. "I felt like I was turning into a prune, I was in the shower so long!" she says. Every time the nurse came in the room looking for the mother, the father hollered: "She'll be right out! Just a little longer." She finally came out of the shower when it was time to push.

I recommend that the father (or other birth partner) help the mother bathe or shower. While the mother is taking a bath, the father can pour water from a glass or pitcher over her abdomen if she finds this helpful. If she is showering, he can stand nearby or shower with her if he prefers. He should bring swim trunks along if the mother is laboring in a hospital or a childbearing center.

Hot compresses can also promote relaxation and ease pain during labor. The birth partner or caregiver can thoroughly wet a hot towel and wring out excess water, then apply it to the area of discomfort, such as the lower back or abdomen. The compresses should be changed often to keep them warm.

Birth in the Water

If the mother chooses to give birth in the water, she will remain in the tub throughout the birth process and sometimes for a short while afterward. The caregiver can monitor labor's progress and the baby's heart tones in the water just as on a labor bed.

Experienced waterbirth midwife Susanna Napierala monitors the fetal heartbeat with a Doptone, a portable stethoscope that emits ultrasound (high-frequency sound waves) that are reflected off the fetal heart and produce echoes that are then translated to the audible sound of the baby's heartbeat. She used to have to ask the mother to raise her hips out of the water so she could place her Doptone on the mother's abdomen, but now she uses a model that can be placed right against the mother's abdomen underwater.

Most mothers deliver in the sit-squat position or on hands and knees. Providing the tank is large enough, the mother is readily able to adopt the position of her choice. For example, when she was pushing, one mother squatted with her husband's support; when the baby's head was crowning, she sat back in the water to give birth.

The physician, midwife, and nurses usually remain outside the tub where they can assist if necessary. However, some practitioners prefer to be right in the tub with the mother. If the tub is sufficiently large, the mother's mate and perhaps others can also join her.

Immediately after birth, the baby is lifted slowly and gently to the surface. In Pithiviers, this is always done within seconds but without any rushing. Just before the baby is brought to the surface, it may open its eyes and look around, unfurling its limbs, while still underwater. When her daughter Halley was born in a homemade redwood tub, Jeannine Parvati, well-known childbirth educator and author of *Prenatal Yoga*, says, "She emerged with open and exploring eyes." Once at the surface, the newborn's breathing is triggered by contact with the air and by the sudden difference in temperature and pressure.

The parents can begin the process of parent–infant bonding in the tub. The mother can hold her child to her breast and begin breastfeeding or just explore her child with her eyes and fingertips. The father too can hold the baby skin-to-skin and enjoy eye contact in the tub.

The baby's body can be kept warm in the water. With the mother's or father's hands on its back for support, the baby can lie back and float. Erika recalls, "After Jason was born, I held him so his face was above water and let him float for about twenty minutes." When it was time for third-stage labor (the delivery of the placenta), she got out of the water and delivered the placenta while semireclining on a bed near the insulated water tank she had used.

As noted previously, it's best to get out of the tub to deliver the placenta to avoid potentially serious complications. It's difficult to monitor the volume of blood loss in the water, and the delivery can be rather messy, since the mother may lose considerable blood with the afterbirth.

Once the umbilical cord is cut, when the mother leaves the tub the baby can still remain in the water with the father, giving the father time to get to know his child. Some mothers return to the tub after the placenta is delivered.

Many women find that waterbirth creates an easier, less painful, and shorter second-stage labor. As one mother put it, "I think the delivery was significantly less painful and exhausting than it might have been 'on land.' I was also able to spread out my energy consumption more easily. I didn't tire myself out."

Dr. Robert Doughton, who has assisted with nearly one hundred waterbirths in Portland, Oregon, points out that warm water contributes to perineal relaxation. "Nothing can better relax the perineum than a body-temperature bath," he says. In addition, as Dr. Odent points out, "Immersion in water seems to help women lose their inhibitions." This can enable the mother to surrender to labor and thereby give birth more efficiently.

"The buoyant weightlessness of floating in the water seemed to lighten the heavy 'bearing down' feeling of contractions," recalls Anne Rivers. "The warm water helped the tissues to stretch." Anne was able to give birth without an episiotomy for the first time. "I could sit down and move around with no pain. What a difference! Recovery was a grand time resting with the baby!"

For the baby, waterbirth is a peaceful beginning to life outside the womb. The baby's transition from the intrauterine environment is made as soft, as gentle, and as peaceful as possible. In addition, the need for oxygen is significantly decreased, because the baby's movements are minimized and body heat is conserved in the warm water. This, some waterbirth proponents claim, decreases stress to the baby's system during the minutes immediately following birth.

In an article entitled "Some Medical Implications Supporting Underwater Birth," Barbara Keller points out that if the umbilical cord has been cut early, the baby's lungs may not be able to supply its total oxygen needs. This possible trauma is eliminated if cord-cutting is delayed or if the baby is born in warm water, where it will require less oxygen. Dr. Charkovsky claims that being protected from the potentially damaging effects of oxygen deprivation after birth, infants born in water are more able to progress steadily and develop more quickly through their first two to four months of life.

Many parents choose waterbirth for the benefits to both the mother and the baby. "I chose a waterbirth because I enjoy the water," Beth says. "When I'm cramped or upset, I often take a bath. So I figured if you're experiencing pain, what better place to be than sitting in water? Then when I began doing research on waterbirth, I found that apart from it being something that was nice for me, waterbirth also provided the baby a much less traumatic entry into the world. It is a beautiful and peaceful way to have a baby."

The Newborn Bath

Immersing the baby in warm water immediately after birth, many parents and professionals believe, significantly reduces birth trauma. The "Leboyer bath," a postnatal warm-water bath, was popularized by the well-known French obstetrician Frederick Leboyer, who advocated a gentle birth process.

Dr. Leboyer's concept of gentle birth consists of several practical rules. First, birth should take place in a quiet place with subdued light. After being in the semidark womb for nine months, the baby's eyes are quite sensitive. If the room is brightly lit, the baby will screw up its eyes to shut out the light. If the lights are subdued, however, parents and baby can enjoy that wonderful experience of eye contact that follows a natural birth. Second, keeping the environment free of unnecessary noise prevents the baby from being rudely shocked after having heard only muted sounds in the womb. Finally, immediately following birth, parents and baby should be together for the bonding process for at least one hour without

BENEFITS OF WATERBIRTH

Laboring women and childbirth professionals have noted the following benefits of labor and giving birth while immersed in warm water.

- Greater maternal relaxation during first- and second-stage labor
- Less pain during labor
- More efficient and more rapid labor
- Perineal relaxation and stretching
- Less traumatic birth
- Enhanced maternal–infant bonding

interuption. All newborn procedures, such as the use of eyedrops to prevent infection, weighing, measuring, and the routine newborn exam, should be delayed.

Unless there is a medical reason to do otherwise, the umbilical cord should be allowed to finish pulsing before it is cut. This way, the baby receives some of the blood still in the placenta. Once the cord is cut, Dr. Leboyer advocates placing the baby in water that has been heated to body temperature. There, in the warm-water bath, the baby will open its eyes and calmly take in the environment, gazing at its parents' faces.

Today the Leboyer bath is commonplace in hospitals throughout the United States. Interestingly, when it was first introduced here, professionals had a similar concern about safety that they now have about waterbirth. Strict sterile technique was employed, including the use of a sterilized stainless-steel basin and sterile water for the bath. Now, however, these unnecessary procedures are no longer observed. Professionals have learned that heated tap water is perfectly fine.

With little doubt, the newborn bath can reduce postbirth trauma, particularly in the clinical environment of the stainless-steel delivery room. However, a gentle birth can be created whether or not the newborn bath is used. Giving birth in a dimly lit, home-like environment and delaying all newborn procedures will accomplish your goals as well. Many parents feel that during the first postnatal hour, the best place for the baby is at its mother's breast or held skin to skin against its father's chest.

It's interesting to note that gentle birth has far-reaching implications and may actually be the beginning of a nonviolent life. After a lengthy investigation of the "roots of crime," the Commission on Crime Control and Violence Prevention in Sacramento, California recommended, among other things, alternative birth including parental involvement, family intimacy, and a natural delivery that discourages overuse of intensive-care nurseries and labor-inducing drugs. Waterbirth midwife Anne Rivers agrees: "For me, waterbirth is more than just a comfortable way to birth a baby. Consciously creating peace for our children from the very moment of birth is the gentle beginning of new possibilities for creating global harmony."

PREPARING FOR WATERBIRTH

"There is nothing mystical about waterbirth," says Dr. Rosenthal. "You don't have to take a special course to enjoy this natural and healthy way to have a baby." However, you should make careful birth plans.

Choose your birth place. Your choices include hospital or childbearing center, home, and perhaps even a warm ocean.

At the present time, there are only a few childbearing centers and hospitals where a woman can have a waterbirth. However, the staff at the childbearing center nearest your home may be willing to consider their first waterbirth if you request one. For a list of the names and addresses of hospitals and childbirth centers where waterbirth occurs, contact Waterbirth International. The name and address of this organization is located in the Resource section at the back of the book.

For most parents who choose waterbirth, home is the only practical birth place. If you plan a home waterbirth, also read Chapter Four for information on preparing for home birth.

A few mothers have given birth in the ocean. One couple traveled to the Bahamas to give birth. The mother labored in the serene tropical water while her husband supported her. Parents who plan to do this should, of course, have an experienced caregiver and make contingency plans in the event of inclement weather.

A marine biologist from Yale University who was the captain of a research ship circumnavigating the waters off the coast of Puerto Rico planned to give birth in the ocean. She had commissioned midwife Susanna Napierala to travel with her to attend the ocean birth. However, labor began before they could find a suitable location. Fortunately, they had previously alerted some friends, who were part of the research team based on land, to prepare a child's wading pool so they would have a backup vessel just in case bad weather or other conditions made ocean birth difficult. This mother ended up giving birth in the wading pool.

One of the most fascinating births Susanna observed was that of a Soviet pediatrician who gave birth in the Black Sea: "Every year in July and August, Igor Charkovsky and his associates from Moscow and Leningrad get together and camp out near the Black Sea," Susanna recalls. "A number of couples including a pediatrician and her husband were waiting to go into labor, and a German midwife and other people, like me, were there to learn more about Igor's methods. The water was only about 80 degrees. And when I knew women were going to be giving birth there, I thought 'Holy Cow! Is this safe?' But apparently births that take place there occur without problems. The mother spent some time laboring on land and some time in the sea. At the time of birth, she assumed a squatting position and her husband caught the baby in the water."

Here are some additional steps to take wherever the birth takes place.

Select a competent caregiver. Though midwives and physicians who have experience with waterbirth are few and far between, a local caregiver may be willing to learn enough about the subject to help you. There is not much difference between assisting a woman to give birth in the water and helping her on a labor bed. Recently when I asked one midwife whether she had ever attended a waterbirth, she said, "No, but I'd love to!" None of her clients had ever requested a waterbirth. So, ask. At the very least, you will have helped acquaint more professionals with this option.

Should your physician or midwife want more information on the subject, Waterbirth International will send educational information at your request.

Develop a positive attitude. A positive view of birth is an essential ingredient in a safe, happy childbearing experience wherever you plan to have the baby. Midwife Anne Rivers recommends examining your feelings and uncovering any possible fears you may have about water as well as examining your feelings about childbirth prior to labor.

Dr. Charkovsky agrees. He believes that a woman's state of mind during pregnancy is of vital importance. For this reason, he works extensively with the mother, using guided-imagery exercises to eliminate her fear of birth and of water. In addition to helping her develop a positive state of mind, he has found that the mother can greatly ease the physical distress of delivery by visualizing the pelvic region expanding and opening. He also suggests imagining the fetus inside the womb surrounded by a golden light.

WATERBIRTH SUPPLIES

For a home waterbirth, most waterbirth practitioners recommend having the following supplies. (See also Chapter Four.)

- A suitable birthing tub, either a fiberglass hot tub, a Jacuzzi, or a bathtub.
- An accurate water thermometer. (The water temperature should be between 99 and 101 degrees F.)
- An underwater flashlight, so the caregiver can view the birth.
- A waterproof watch, to time contractions if necessary and to note the time of birth.
- An inflatable plastic pillow.
- A strainer or fish net to catch any floating debris.
- Several towels.

The Birth Tub

In the United States, a wide variety of containers have been used for waterbirth. These include a fiberglass hot tub, a Jacuzzi, a standard-sized bathtub, a children's wading pool, several types of homemade birthing tanks, and even a steel watering trough.

For the birth of their child, Nancy and her husband, Gaston, set up an eight-foot-diameter child's wading pool in their immaculately heated basement. Waterbed heaters kept the water at the right temperature (99 to 101 degrees Fahrenheit).

Another couple, Beth and Jacques, set up a rented portable tank on the second floor of their Victorian home for the birth of their daughter, Dominique. "The tank had four wooden side panels that fit together and a plastic liner," says Beth. "The sides had heating panels in them to keep the water at a certain temperature. The drawback of having to set up a portable tank," she points out, "is that you have to keep the tank sterile and keep changing the water every three days until you go into labor. But in my situation, the baby was born the day we put up the tub so we didn't have to worry about changing water."

Dr. Jan-Erik Strole, who has recently begun doing waterbirths at St. Joseph's Hospital in Polsen, Montana, uses a large Jacuzzi tub.

A few parents have built their own birthing tubs. For instance, when Jeannine Parvati was pregnant with her sixth child, Halley, her husband, Rico, built a deep redwood tub where Jeannine gave birth enclosed in a glass greenhouse.

Dissatisfied with available tanks, Jeff Rene, a fine woodworker in Windsor, California, built his own tank for the birth of his two children. "We wanted a clean environment we could control," he says. "In addition, we wanted something comfortable and convenient." Since the waterbirths of his children, he has been designing waterbirth tanks for others.

If you use a Jacuzzi or whirlpool for waterbirth, the power should be off at the time of the birth. Also, remember that Jacuzzi jets have filter systems that are difficult to clean.

Parents can also rent portable, inflatable birthing tubs from Waterbirth International. Their tubs can be shipped anywhere in the United States.

The Water

The water temperature should be between 99 and 101 degrees Fahrenheit. It is also essential that the water to be used during labor is clean. Linda Church of The Family Birthing Center in Upland says: "We ensure that the tub is bacteria free by taking bacterial cultures at least weekly. After each use, the tubs are thoroughly scrubbed with detergent and sterilized." However, the water is ordinary tap water and contains no chemical additives. In Pithiviers also, the water is not sterilized and contains no chemicals or additives of any kind. If the mother releases a small amount of feces into the water during second-stage labor (which is common wherever birth takes place), it is removed with a net.

Once labor has begun, there is no way to keep the water bacteria free. However, bear in mind that childbirth is not a sterile process. Sensible personal hygiene is adequate to ensure a clean birth environment.

LOOKING AHEAD

My hope is that more practitioners will learn about waterbirth and that this childbirth option will become more widely available. We need more practitioners like Linda Ford, who was willing to learn about waterbirth to help a client create the birth she desired, and Susanna Napierala, who researched waterbirth because a couple said it was their chosen birth method.

The future of waterbirth depends largely on educating health practitioners about the benefits of using water throughout the childbearing process. But fulfilling, joyful waterbirths depend on more than merely realizing that the method is safe and installing hot tubs in hospitals. What is most needed is a change in the approach—a shift from the attempt to control labor to the willingness to surrender to it. Such a change rests on the ability of practitioners—physicians, midwives, nurses, and childbirth educators—to accept birth as a natural process.

Most important of all, the future of waterbirth depends on the consumers. Speaking of waterbirth becoming more readily available, Dr. Rosenthal says: "There is only one way it's going to happen. It won't come from universities; it won't come from doctors; it will come from consumers, that is, mothers and fathers. As more birthing places offer waterbirth as an option, women will walk away from doctors who say 'No.' The establishment will be forced to change due to consumer demand."

It is of the utmost importance that parents be free to choose the kind of birth they want and for you, the mother, to be free to give birth in the position you feel most comfortable, whether that be squatting on your bedroom floor, lying on a hospital labor bed, or relaxing in a tank filled with warm water.

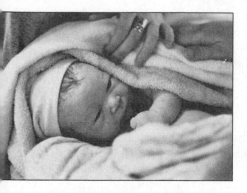

For Us
to Create

IN MANY WAYS, WE ARE EMERG-
ing from an obstetric dark age. Healthy, rewarding options for
mother and baby are slowly replacing the dehumanizing maternity
care of the past. As more and more parents choose home birth,
childbearing-center birth, birth in hospitals with a positive emotional climate, waterbirth, and midwifery care, these options will
eventually be considered the norm rather than "alternatives."

For now, however, there is much room for improvement. Home-
birth services are not available everywhere, and in many childbearing centers screening requirements are still overly rigid, preventing
hundreds of healthy mothers from giving birth within their doors.
Although hospitals are improving, institutions with all the characteristics described in Chapter Seven are few and far between. In
many areas, certified nurse-midwives are not granted hospital privileges, and direct-entry midwives do not yet have hospital privileges anywhere. Many nurse-midwives will not attend home
births. And unless they live close to one of the very few centers in
the world where waterbirth is practiced, most parents must go to
great lengths to prepare for this option.

The conventional medical approach in the United States today
has had a virtual monopoly on health care since the 1800s.
However, this is changing. People are beginning to realize that
other methods of health care including homeopathy, chiropractic
medicine, and acupuncture are safe and effective. The alternative-

birth movement cannot be separated from the widespread trend toward recognizing other methods of health care. Eventually some of the concepts underlying the alternative-birth philosophy, such as the view that labor is a normal and natural event, not an illness, will no doubt replace traditional views of labor.

Yet alternative birth is still in its newborn period. If it is to grow and survive, dramatic changes must be made in the way many professionals view childbirth. As David Stewart, PhD, of NAPSAC points out, the current maternal/child-health care system is seriously flawed. It cannot simply be modified but requires several fundamental changes.

First, we need to adopt a new model of childbirth that encompasses the laboring mother's psychological, emotional, and behavioral as well as physiological changes. I have outlined such a model, which I call the laboring mind response, in Chapter Two.

Second, we need major changes in legislation, granting parents freedom of choice in childbirth. This means that direct-entry as well as certified nurse-midwives must be allowed to practice through-out the United States. The major medical organizations also need legislation forbidding hospitals and other physicians from revoking a practitioner's privileges because he or she attends a home birth. Parents do not have the freedom to choose childbirth options when practitioners who attend home births are punished in this way.

Third, we need many more publicized studies to prove that alternative-birth methods are safe. The major areas that need more research are the safety of home birth, the safety of childbearing-center birth, and the advantages of waterbirth. Thousands of health professionals remain ignorant of the impressive safety statistics associated with these options. Advocates of alternative birth know that being in an emotionally positive environment can lead to a more efficient labor; however, it is important to prove this statistically. We also need to measure the effects of guided imagery on the mother's experience of labor and prove what health professionals who have used the method know from experience: that guided imagery reduces fear, pain, the length of labor, and the likelihood of a cesarean.

WHAT YOU CAN DO

You can help shape the future of childbirth. Readers who are alarmed at the national cesarean rate, who are disturbed by unfair laws discriminating against midwifery care, or who are disappointed about the lack of options for alternative-birth methods in their area can work toward change. Many expectant and new parents become childbirth activists working for change in their community.

If you would like to see the childbirth options discussed in this book become more widely available in your area, you can take any of several steps.

Apply consumer pressure. Pressure from consumers often helps to trigger change, particularly in hospitals. If you are dissatisfied with the hospitals in your area, write to hospital administrators and let them know why you will not (or did not) give birth in their institutions. Or, if you have had a disappointing birth experience in a hospital, let administrators know about it. If enough people express dissatisfaction with rigid policies, lack of midwife services, inadequate backup for home-birth services, and overly interventive obsteric care, change is more likely to occur.

Set up educational programs for parents and health professionals. Invite a health professional to plan a workshop educating parents and other professionals about their options in your area. Education alone is sometimes enough to trigger major breakthroughs. In addition, planning a workshop can give your cause effective local publicity. It can generate radio, TV, and newspaper publicity for alternative-birth methods, making health-care consumers aware of their choices.

If you would like to set up an alternative-birth workshop in your area, see the section entitled "Workshops" in the Resources at the back of this book.

Organize a childbirth group. A group of parents and professionals working together can educate health-care consumers, disseminate information about alternative birth, and perhaps even lobby for legislative change in midwifery laws. The InterNational Association of Parents and Professionals for Safe Alternatives in Childbirth (NAPSAC), which now has member groups throughout the world, began with seven people: two couples, two mothers, and a health-care professional. NAPSAC can give you some guidelines in starting your own group. Their address and phone number are listed in the Resources at the back of this book.

Get publicity for alternative-birth methods. Present information on the safety and benefits of childbirth alternatives on the agenda at public health meetings, before the board of trustees at publicly funded hospitals, and at hospital childbirth classes, health fairs, conferences, and any other meeting or organization associated with childbirth.

Take responsibility for your own birth. This is the single most important step to take in inspiring change. I often hear mothers make remarks like "the physician allowed me to get up and walk around during labor," or "the hospital allowed my mother to remain with us during the birth." Remember, it's *your* birth and *your* baby, not the physician's or hospital's. Your caregiver is someone *you* hire. By taking responsibility for your own birth, it is more likely that you will have a rewarding and fulfilling as well as safe, healthy birth.

Many believe that physicians are responsible for shaping the future of childbirth, as they are the ones who design the procedures. Others believe that hospitals, who write the policies, are responsible. Some look to legislators, who make the laws.

However, the future of childbirth does not lie with any of these people. It is we, the parents, who will determine the changes that will be made. Ultimately, childbirth reflects our relationship with nature, our feelings about our bodies, our attitudes about sexuality, and our beliefs about birth. We shape our own birth experiences by what we believe about birth and by the choices we make.

The future of childbirth is for us to create.

Notes

Chapter 1
Giving Birth Your Way

2 "70 percent of all births" G. Marsden Wagner, "Infant Mortality," 473–84.
9 "medical interventions that would not have been required in their homes" Stanley Sagov, *Home Birth*, 23. 10 "decrease the incidence of fetal distress" Y. Liu, "Position During Labor and Delivery." 90 "in the squatting, as compared to the supine, position" J. Russell, "The Rationale of Primitive Delivery Positions," 712–15. 77 "constriction of the mother's blood vessels" Joyce Roberts, "Alternative positions for childbirth." 17 "the worst position for labor and birth" Roberto Caldeyro-Barcia, "Supine called position worst position." 13 "hinders the bearing-down process" J. Caire, "Are Current Rates of Cesarean Justified?" 12 "less than 4 percent requested analgesia" Family Birth Centers, "Current Statistics." 13 "cesarean section rates of less than 10 percent." G. Marsden Wagner, "Infant Mortality," 473–84. 14 "actually may increase the possibility of infection" H. Kantor, "Value of Shaving the Pudendal-Perineal Area." 15 "benefit of electronic fetal monitoring to low-risk patients" National Institutes of Health, *Antenatal Diagnostics.* 15 "double among electronically monitored mothers" I. Kelso, "An Assessment of Continuous Fetal Heart Rate Monitoring," 526–32. 15 "In an often-quoted study" A. Haverkamp, "The Evaluation of Continuous Fetal Heart Rate Monitoring." 16 "correlation between use of EFM and increased cesareans" L. Gilstrap, "Cesarean Section"; R. Paul, "Clinical Fetal Monitoring"; J. Caire, "Are Current Rates of Cesarean Justified?" 16 "observed with the continuously monitored group" Kirkwood K. Shy, "Effects of Electronic Fetal-Heart-Rate Monitoring." 16 "because of the use of noisy, incomprehensible machines" H. Minkoff and R. Schwartz, "The Rising Cesarean Section Rate." 17 "oxygen deprivation from compression of the umbilical cord" K. Baumgarten, "Advantages and disadvantages of low amniotomy," 3–11. 17 "often results in a cesarean" F. Kubli, "Influence of Labor," 168–91; J. Lumley and C. Wood, "Transient Fetal Acidosis," 221–25. 17 "results of this procedure are at best inconsistent and unpredictable" E. Friedman and M. Sachtelben, "Amniotomy and the Course of La-

bor," 755–70. 17 "associated with poor outcome for the offspring" R. Caldeyro-Barcia, "Adverse Perinatal Effects." 19 "increase in the incidence of jaundice in the newborn" A. A. Calder, V. A. Moar, M. K. Oumstead, and A. C. Turnbull, "Increased Bilirubin Levels." 19 "possibly even death" T. H. Booth and V. B. Kurdyak, 245. 19 "episiotomies performed by the majority of U.S. obstetricians" David Banta and Stephen Thacker, "The risks and benefits of episiotomies," 25–30. 22 "no option but to room in with their infants" A. McBride, "Compulsory Rooming-in," 625. 22 "to gain more weight, and to be breastfed longer" M. Klaus and J. H. Kennell, "Mothers Separated from Their Newborn Infants," 1015–37. 22 "enhanced by home birth" G. Peterson, unpublished manuscript, 179. 22 "separated from their parents shortly after birth" C. R. Barnet, "Neonatal Separation," 197; M. H. Klaus and J. H. Kennell, *Maternal-Infant Bonding*. 22 "interfere with the parent–infant attachment process" M. H. Klaus and J. H. Kennell, *Maternal-Infant Bonding*. 24 "separated from her family and her baby" Helen Varney, *Nurse-Midwifery*, 353. 26 "new level of optimism across the land" Elizabeth Hosford, "The Home Birth Movement," 29–30.

Chapter 2
A Safer, More Positive Labor

36 "previously noted by other childbirth professionals" Niles Newton, *Maternal Emotions*. 42 "on recognition of her as a unique individual" Bianca Gorden, *The Place of Birth*, 201.

Chapter 4
Midwifery Care

34. 94 "aware of what exactly nurse-midwifery was" *Nurse-Midwifery in America*; 116. 96. "infant-mortality rate for 1987 was 10.5 per thousand" Deborah A. Sullivan and Rose Weitz, *Labor Pains*, 112–31. 97 "cesarean-section rate was 1.5 percent" Ina May Gaskin, *Spiritual Midwifery*, 474–75. 98 "results as good as this one run by midwives" David Stewart, "The Five Standards," 122–23. 98 "more than tripled, to 32.1 per thousand!" T. Montgomery, "A Case for Nurse-Midwives," 50–58 99 "proposed that midwives' hospital privileges be increased" Institute of Medicine, "Prenatal Care." 100 "(primarily resulting from the use of forceps)" L. Mehl, "Research on Alternatives," 171–207. 103 "debased their character as well" Ernest L. Boyer, "Midwifery in America," 1. 103 "physicians were gentlemen whose hands were clean" Richard W. Wertz and Dorothy C. Wertz, *Lying-In*, 119–24. 104 "disappearance of a centuries-old profession . . . was no accident" David Stewart, "The Five Standards," 112.

Chapter 5
Birth At Home

110. "the worst hospital settings may increase obstetric casualties" Stanley Sagov, *Home Birth*. 110 "less need for infant resuscitation" Lewis Mehl, "Evaluation of

outcomes," 17–29. 111 "from anesthetized hospital to home delivery" G. H. Peterson, "Effects of Childbirth," 114. 111 "five times greater in out-of-hospital than in hospital birth" American College of Obstetricians and Gynecologists, "Health department data." 111 "study published in the *American Journal of Obstetrics and Gynecology* gives similar statistics" Kirkwood Shy, Floyd Frost, and Jean Ullom, "Out-of-hospital delivery," 547–52. 172 "associated with increased perinatal mortality" M. Hinds, Gershom Bergeisen, and David Allen, "Neonatal outcomes," 1578–82. 112 "calling themselves midwives" Lewis Mehl, "Evaluation of outcomes," 17–29. 113 "this very small but real risk . . . incurred in the hospital" Stanley Sagov, *Home Birth*, 33. 120 "keenly interested and highly motivated" Elizabeth Hosford, "Alternative Patterns." 120 "responsibility for their own and their children's health care" Lester D. Hazell, "A study of 300 elective home births," 11–18; Lewis Mehl and Gail H. Peterson, "Home birth versus hospital birth"; Carolyn Searles, "The impetus toward home birth." 126 "if the pregnancy is normal and the baby is healthy" Tonya Brooks, "Unattended Home Births," 518. 126 "hospital neonatal death rate was seven per thousand" Claude A. Burnett III, "Home Delivery," 2741–45. 126 "we decided to do it ourselves" Tonya Brooks, "Unattended Home Births," 518. 128 "delayed onset . . . beyond forty-two weeks' gestation" Deborah A. Sullivan and Rose Weitz, *Labor Pains*, 112–32. 132 " . . . the fault will be called yours!" Lester D. Hazell, *Commonsense Childbirth*, 190. 133 Deborah A. Sullivan and Rose Weitz, *Labor Pains*, 142. " . . . if my malpractice insurance wasn't $23,000."

Chapter 6
Birth in a childbearing center

144 "Only secondarily is childbirth seen as a medical event" Pamela S. Eakins, "Women and Health," 53. 145 "education, motivation, and support provided women in labor" Carla Reinke, "Outcomes of the First 527 Births," 238. 146 "more important . . . than any other single factor" M. E. Hosford, "Implementing a Medically Sound Childbearing Center," 311. 154 "less than half that for mothers in the hospital (14 percent)" A. Sculphome; A. G. McLeod; E. G. Robertson, "A Birth Center Affiliated with the Tertiary Care Center," 589–603. 157 "an indication for obstetric management is an indication for transfer" J. B. Faison, "The Childbearing Center."

Chapter 7
Hospital Birth

164 "increased from three in 1975 to over 120 in 1982" L. L. Ostrowsky, *Alternative Birth Centers*. 165 "68 percent . . . compared to 16 percent of home-birth mothers" Aidan Macfarlane, *The Psychology of Childbirth*. 171 "no difference in labor options between hospitals with and without birthing rooms" Raymond DeVries, "Image and Reality," 3–9. 173 "private-patient deliveries increased 126 percent" J. Kell Williams and Mathew R. Mervis, "Use of the labor-delivery-recovery room," 23–24. 184 " . . . obvious to the family just who is in charge, i.e., the professional staff" Susan McKay and Celeste R. Phillips, "Family Centered

Maternity Care," 4. 187 "regardless of the specifics of the birth experience" Ibid., 51. 190 "family centered birthing environment within the hospital setting" *Bulletin of the New York Academy of Medicine*, 401–02.

Chapter 8
Waterbirth

194 "these same women will . . . not want to leave!" Michel Odent, *Birth Reborn*, 46. 199 "has only known watery environments" Ibid., 50. 199 "He's never done anything else." Ibid., 50. 200 "oxygenation of the fetal blood that is being brought to the placenta decreases immediately" Rosenthal, Michael, *Pre- and Perinatal Psychology News*, 20. 200 "must be immediately lifted to the air to breathe" *Journal of Nurse Midwifery*, 168. 200 "amazingly simple intervention of allowing a woman to sit in warm water" *Pre- and Perinatal Psychology News*, 22. 202 "the direct muscular stretching action; and peripheral vascular action" *Lancet*, Sidenbladh 84 [msp 331—Maidstone quote not indicated in ms] *Midwives' Chronicle and Nursing Notes*, 289. 204 "I didn't tire myself out." Eric Sidenbladh, *Water Babies*, 92. 207 "gentle beginning of new possibilities for creating global harmony" Anne Rivers, *Gentle Beginnings*, 11. 210 "tubs are thoroughly scrubbed with detergent and sterilized" *Journal of Nurse-Midwifery*, 166.

Resources

ORGANIZATIONS

Alternatives in Childbirth

The InterNational Association for Parents and Professionals for Safe Alternatives in Childbirth (NAPSAC)
Route 1, Box 646
Marble HIll, Missouri 63764
(314) 238-2010

NAPSAC publishes books and pamphlets supporting alternative birth. The organization also publishes a *Directory of Alternative Birth Services and Consumer Guide*. There are NAPSAC member groups throughout the world. Write for a list.

Breastfeeding

Natural Technologies Inc./White River
23010 Lake Forest Drive, Suite 310
Laguna Hills, California 92653
1(800) 824-6351

White River makes the only breast pump that has been medically proven to produce serum prolactin levels (the *mothering* hormone associated with milk production) equivalent to the needs of a nursing baby. It also maintains a twenty-four-hour breastfeeding hotline to answer questions and offer assistance with breastfeeding.

La Leche League, International (LLLI)
9616 Minneapolis Avenue
Franklin Park, Illinois 60131
(708) 455-7730
1 (800) 525-3243 [1(800) LA-LECHE]

This international organization provides information about and support for breastfeeding both over the telephone and in local neighborhood meetings. LLLI also publishes many informative pamphlets and books. Write or call for a complete list.

Specially trained persons called "leaders," who are located in most major cities throughout the United States and Europe, provide breastfeeding information. Try the telephone directory for the name of the La Leche League leader in your area. If there is no listing, call the national office for information.

Other nursing mothers' groups. There are many smaller nursing mothers' support groups throughout the world. Some childbirth-education organizations have their own nursing mothers' counselors. Local childbirth educators, childbearing centers, and some maternity hospitals may be able to give you a local reference.

Childbirth Education

The childbirth educators associated with the following organizations teach a wide variety of methods. They may have strikingly different approaches from one another. For this reason, it is essential to interview a childbirth educator on an individual basis before making a decision whether or not to take his or her classes.

International Childbirth Education Association (ICEA)
P.O. Box 20048
Minneapolis, Minnesota 55420
(612) 854-8660

This organization certifies childbirth educators and distributes information about childbirth. Contact the national office for the name of a childbirth educator in your area.

The American Society for Psychoprophylaxis in Obstetrics (ASPO)
1840 Wilson Boulevard, Suite 204
Arlington, Virginia 22201
(800) 368-4404

This organization, which introduced the Lamaze method to the United States, certifies childbirth educators. Contact the national office for the name of a childbirth educator in your area.

Informed Homebirth/Informed Birth and Parenting
P.O. Box 3675
Ann Arbor, Michigan 48106
(313) 662-6857

This organization certifies childbirth educators who prepare parents to make well-informed decisions regardless of the place of birth. Contact the national office for a childbirth educator in your area.

The Academy of Certified Childbirth Educators
(800) 444-8223

This organization certifies childbirth educators throughout the United States. Contact the national office for a childbirth educator in your area.

Cesarean Prevention

Cesarean/Support, Education & Concern (C/SEC)
22 Forest Road
Framingham, Massachusetts 01701
(617) 877-8266

C/Sec provides information on cesarean prevention and vaginal birth after cesarean as well as support for cesarean families through telephone and person-to-person contact.

Cesarean Prevention Movement (CPM)
P.O. Box 152, University Station
Syracuse, New York 13210
(315) 424-1942

CPM offers information on and support for cesarean prevention and vaginal birth after cesarean. There are many CPM chapters throughout the country. Write or call for the chapter nearest your home.

Childbearing Centers

National Association of Childbearing Centers (NACC)
RFD 1, Box 1
Perkiomenville, Pennsylvania 18074
(215) 234-8068

This organization will provide the names and addresses of childbearing centers throughout the United States. (Enclose a self-addressed stamped envelope.)

High-Risk Pregnancy and Unexpected Outcomes

Intensive Caring Unlimited (ICU)
910 Bent Lane
Philadelphia, Pennsylvania 19118
(215) 233-4723

ICU provides support and resources for parents of premature or hospitalized babies, those with developmental delays, parents experiencing high-risk pregnancy, and those whose babies have died.

Parent Care Inc.
101 ½ South Union
Alexandria, Virginia 22314-3323
(703) 836-4678

This organization provides support and references for parents with
high-risk pregnancy, parents of premature or hospitalized babies,
and parents whose babies have died. Call for a reference to a parent
support group in your area.

Coping with Loss

The Compassionate Friends
P.O. Box 1347
Oak Brook, Illinois 60521
(708) 990-0010

This organization, with chapters throughout the world, provides
support and encouragement for parents who have lost a child. Call
the national office for a local reference.

Waterbirth

Waterbirth International
P.O. Box 5554
Santa Barbara, California 93150
(800) 565-3980

This organization provides educational literature and videos about
waterbirth.

Workshops

I am currently conducting four workshops to educate both parents
and childbirth professionals about the options in this book:

Alternative Birth, a practical discussion of alternative-birth
options in the hospital, childbearing center, and home, including

waterbirth and midwifery care, focusing on the safety and benefits of these childbirth methods.

Mind Over Labor, a highly practical approach to childbirth education and coping with labor based on understanding the psychological changes of the laboring mother and on using guided imagery.

The Father's Role During Pregnancy, Birth, and Beyond, an approach to educating and actively involving fathers as well as meeting the father's needs through pregnancy, labor, and the postpartum period.

Prenatal Intuition, a discussion of the wide variety of intuitive experiences common during pregnancy, the practical value of paying attention to intuition, and ways to enhance one's own intuitive abilities.

Some other childbirth professionals have workshops that educate parents and professionals about alternative-birth options. Contact your local childbirth educator for information.

SUGGESTED READING

Pregnancy and Childbirth

Pregnancy, Childbirth, and the Newborn: A Complete Guide for Expectant Parents, by Penny Simkin, Janet Whalley, and Ann Keppler (Deephaven, MN: Meadowbrook, 1984, $10.95). An easy-to-use, thorough, up-to-date guide to a healthy pregnancy and newborn, this book covers exercise, prenatal nutrition, the advantages and disadvantages of obstetric interventions including medication, and feeding the baby.

The Well Pregnancy Book, by Mike Samuels, M.D., and Nancy Samuels (New York: Summit, 1986, $14.95). This book is a comprehensive guide to prenatal health and medical information for expectant parents.

Pregnancy and Dreams, by Patricia Maybruck, PhD (Los Angeles: Jeremy Tarcher, 1989, $10.95). This fascinating account of the dream world of pregnancy will enable the mother to have a more peaceful pregnancy by understanding her dreams, fantasies, and nightmares.

Guided Imagery in Pregnancy and Labor

Mind Over Labor, by Carl Jones (New York: Viking/Penguin, 1987, $7.95). This concise guide, which introduced the method of guided imagery to the childbearing public, shows how the mind influences labor. It offers simple exercises to enjoy a healthier, happier pregnancy; reduce the fear and pain of labor; reduce the chance of complications, including fetal distress, and of having a cesarean section; and enable expectant parents to prepare for a safe, positive birth experience.

Visualizations for an Easier Childbirth, by Carl Jones (Deephaven, MN: Meadowbrook, 1989, $5.95). This book is a collection of thirty-five guided-imagery and relaxation exercises to enable expectant parents to enjoy a healthier, lower-stress pregnancy and a shorter, more relaxed labor.

Labor Support

Birth Partner's Handbook, by Carl Jones (Deephaven, MN: Meadowbrook, 1988, $5.95). An easy-to-understand guide that provides step-by-step instructions for comforting and helping the laboring woman from the first contractions to the first days after birth, this book is for fathers or anyone planning to help a mother through labor.

Sharing Birth: A Father's Guide to Giving Support During Labor, by Carl Jones (Granby, MA: Bergin & Garvey, 1989, $12.95). This guide to providing labor support is addressed to the father (or other birth partner) who wants to be as well-informed as possible. It covers everything the birth partner should know about reducing the fear and pain of labor and helping the mother make a smooth beginning to the first few days of new parenthood.

The Postpartum Period

After the Baby Is Born, by Carl Jones (New York: Henry Holt, 1988, $8.95). Addressing *both* parents, this postpartum guide shows how to make the transition to new parenthood as smooth as possible. It covers reducing postpartum blues, relieving common physical discomforts, getting back in shape, making love after birth, and hastening recovery after a cesarean birth.

The New Mother Care, by Lynn DelliQuadri and Kati Breckenridge (Los Angeles: Jeremy Tarcher, 1978, $6.95). This postpartum guide shows the mother how to help herself through the emotional transitions of new parenthood.

The Newborn

The Well Baby Book, by Mike Samuels, M.D., and Nancy Samuels (New York: Summit, 1979, $12.95). This comprehensive manual covers baby care, from conception to age four.

Babies Remember Birth, by David Chamberlain, PhD (Los Angeles: Jeremy Tarcher, 1988, $16.95). This fascinating book discusses extraordinary scientific discoveries about the mind and personality of the newborn. It includes breakthrough evidence showing that babies remember their own birth and sometimes even prenatal experiences, as well as practical information about making your baby's early memories the best possible.

For Fathers

The Birth of a Father, by Martin Greenberg, M.D. (New York: Avon, 1985, $3.95). A moving account of a man's transition to fatherhood, this book explores the sense of absorption, fascination, and love a father feels for his new child.

When Men Are Pregnant, by Jerrold Lee Shapiro, PhD (San Luis Obispo, CA: Impact, 1987, $8.95). A trimester-by-trimester exploration of pregnancy for men, this book discusses the needs and concerns of expectant fathers.

Children at Birth

Mom and Dad and I Are Having a Baby!, by Maryann P. Malecki, R.N. (Seattle, WA: Pennypress, 1982, $6.95). A well-illustrated book for children about childbirth, this simple guide gives a child everything he or she needs to know to attend a sibling's birth.

Cesarean Prevention

Birth Without Surgery: A Guide to Preventing Unnecessary Cesareans and Preparing for Vaginal Birth After Cesarean, by Carl

Jones (Granby, MA: Bergin & Garvey, 1990). This guide gives parents practical steps to reduce the chance of a cesarean and prepare for VBAC (vaginal birth after cesarean).

Silent Knife, by Nancy Wainer Cohen and Lois J. Estner (Granby, MA: Bergin & Garvey, 1983, $14.95). A powerful and factual exposé, about the rising U.S. cesarean rate and its causes, this book has hundreds of references to medical articles regarding the dangers of cesarean birth and medical interventions.

Childbirth Alternatives

The NAPSAC guides are invaluable references, including the summaries of thousands of medical articles documenting the safety of alternative-birth methods and the dangers of conventional obstetric interventions. They include:

The Five Standards of Safe Childbearing, by David Stewart, PhD (Marble Hill, MO: NAPSAC Reproductions, 1981).

21st Century Obstetrics Now, vols. I and II, David Stewart, PhD, and Lee Stewart, editors ($12.95).

Compulsory Hospitalization: Freedom of Choice in Childbirth?, vols. I, II, and III, Stewart and Stewart, editors.

Safe Alternatives in Childbirth, by David Stewart, PhD (Marble Hill, MO: NAPSAC Reproductions, $8.95).

Home Birth

Special Delivery: The Complete Guide to Informed Birth, by Rahima Baldwin (Berkeley, CA: Celestial Arts, 1979, $10.95). A comprehensive, practical guide for parents wanting to give birth at home, this book covers prenatal care and risk screening, nutrition and exercise, care of the newborn, and postdelivery care of the mother.

Midwifery

Hearts and Hands: A Midwife's Guide to Pregnancy and Birth, by Elizabeth Davis (Berkeley, CA: Celestial Arts, 1987, $14.95). This comprehensive, up-to-date guide to midwifery and home birth is for parents as well as professionals.

The Midwife's Pregnancy and Childbirth Book, by Marion McCarney, CNM, and Antonia van der Meer (New York: Henry Holt, 1990, $19.95). A reassuring guide to a healthy pregnancy and safe delivery from a midwife's point of view.

Spiritual Midwifery, by Ina May Gaskin (Summertown, TN: The Book Publishing, 1977, $12.95). A collection of memorable stories of women who gave birth at The Farm, a spiritual/agricultural community in Summertown, Tennessee, this book contains some of the most impressive childbearing statistics ever published.

Miscellaneous

From Parent to Child: The Psychic Link, by Carl Jones (New York: Warner, 1989, $8.95). This book explores the well-documented ESP connection between parent and child. Two chapters are devoted to intuition during pregnancy, and a third chapter covers extrasensory experiences during the early newborn period. The final chapters provide practical exercises for enhancing intuition.

Women's Intuition, by Elizabeth Davis (Berkeley, CA: Celestial Arts, 1989, $7.95). A discussion of the special role intuition plays in women's lives including during the childbearing season, this book suggests various ways in which it can be developed.

NOTE: Many of the books above are available from Naturpath, 1410 N.W. 13th Street, Gainesville, Florida 32601; 1 (800) 542-4784.

Bibliography

American College of Obstetricians and Gynecologists. "Health department data shows danger of home births." January 4, 1978.

Banta, David, and Stephen Thacker. "The risks and benefits of episiotomies: A review." *Birth*, vol. 8 (1982).

Barnet, C. R., et al. "Neonatal Separation: The Maternal Side of Interactional Deprivation." *Pediatrics*, vol. 54 (1970).

Baumgarten, K. "Advantages and disadvantages of low amniotomy." *Journal of Perinatal Medicine*, vol. 4 (1976).

Booth, T. H., and V. B. Kurdyak. 1970. *Canadian Medical Association Journal*, vol. 103.

Boyer, Ernest O. "Midwifery in America: A Profession Reaffirmed." The Carnegie Foundation, May 22, 1990.

Brooks, Tonya. "Unattended Home Births." *Compulsory Hospitalization or Freedom of Choice in Childbirth*, Stewart & Stewart, eds., vol. 11. Marble Hill, MO: NAPSAC Publications, 1979.

Bulletin of the New York Academy of Medicine, vol. 59, no. 4 (May 1983).

Burnett, Claude A. III, et al. "Home Delivery and Neonatal Mortality in North Carolina." *JAMA*, vol. 224, no. 24.

Caire, J. "Are Current Rates of Cesarean Justified?" *Southern Medical Journal*, vol. 71, no. 5 (May 1978).

Calder, A. A.; V. A. Moar; M. K. Oumstead; and A. C. Turnbull. "Increased Bilirubin Levels in Neonates after Induction of Labour by Intravenous Prostaglandins or Oxytocin." *Lancet*, vol. II (1974).

Caldeyro-Barcia, R., et al. "Adverse Perinatal Effects of Early Amniotomy During Labor." *Modern Perinatal Medicine*, L. Gluck, ed. Chicago: Year Book Publishers, 1974.

Caldeyro-Barcia, Roberto. "Supine called worst position during labor and delivery." *Obstetrics and Gynecology News*, June 1975.

Church, Linda. 1989. *Journal of Nurse-Midwifery*, vol. 34, no. 4.

DeVries, Raymond. "Image and Reality: An Evaluation of Hospital Alternative Birth Centers." *Journal of Nurse-Midwifery*, vol. 28 (1983).

Eakins, Pamela S. "Women and Heath." [journal?], vol. 9. no. 4[4?] (Winter 1984).

Faison, J. B., et al. "The Childbearing Center: An Alternative Birth Setting." *Obstetrics and Gynecology*, vol. 54, no. 4 (October 1979).

Family Birth Center. "Current Statistics from January 22, 1979 through December 31, 1989." Providence Hospital, Southfield, MI.

Friedman, E., and M. Sachtelben. "Amniotomy and the Course of Labor." *Obstetrics and Gynecology*, vol. 22 (1963).

Gaskin, Ina May. *Spiritual Midwifery*. Summertown, TN: Book Publishing, 1978.

Gilstrap, L.; J. Hauth; and S. Toussaint. "Cesarean Section: Changing Incidence and Indications." *Obstetrics and Gynecology*, vol. 63, no. 2. (February 1984).

Gordon, Bianca. Article in *The Place of Birth*, Kitzinger and David, eds. New York: Oxford University Press, 1978.

Haverkamp, A., et al. "The Evaluation of Continuous Fetal Heart Rate in Monitoring High-Risk Pregnancy." *American Journal of Obstetrics and Gynecology*, vol. 1, no. 3 (June 1976.

Hazell, Lester D. "A study of 300 elective home births." *Birth and the Family Journal*, vol. 2 (1975).

Hinds, M. Ward; Geshom Bergeisen; and David Allen. "Neonatal outcomes in planned vs. unplanned out-of-hospital births in Kentucky." *Journal of the American Medical Association*, vol. 253.

Hosford, Elizabeth. "Alternative Patterns in Nurse-Midwifery Care." *Journal of Nurse-Midwifery*, vol. 21, no. 3 (1976).

Hosford, Elizabeth, CNM. "The Home Birth Movement." *Journal of Nurse-Midwifery*, vol. 21, no. 3 (1976).

Hosford, M.E. "Implementing a Medically Sound Childbearing Center: Problems and Solutions." In *21st Century Obstetrics*, vol. 3. Marble Hill, MO: NAPSAC Publications, 1977.

Institute of Medicine. *Prenatal Care: Reaching Mothers, Reaching Infants*, Sara S. Brown, ed. Washington, D.C.: National Academy Press, 1988.

Kantor, H., et al. "Value of Shaving the Pudendal-Perineal Area in Delivery Preparation." *Obstetrics and Gynecology*, vol. 25 (1965).

Kelso, I., et al. "An Assessment of Continuous Fetal Heart Rate Monitoring in High-Rish Pregnancy." *American Journal of Obstetrics and Gynecology*, vol. 131, no. 5 (1978).

Klaus, M., and J. H. Kennell. "Mothers Separated from Their Newborn Infants." *Pediatric Clinics of North America*, vol. 17 (1970).

Kubli, F. "Influence of Labor on Fetal Acid-Base Balance." *Clinical Obstetrics and Gynecology*, vol. 11 (1968).

Liu, Y. "Position During Labor and Delivery: History and Perspective." *Journal of Nurse-Midwifery*, vol. 24, no. 3 (May/June 1979).

Lumley, J., and C. Wood. "Transient Fetal Acidosis and Artificial Rupture of the Membranes." *Aust. NZ Journal of Obstetrics and Gynecology*, vol. 11 (1971).

Lynaugh, Kathleen H. "The effects of early elective amniotomy on the length of labor and the condition of the fetus." *Journal of Nurse-Midwifery*, vol. 25 (1980).

Macfarlane, Aidan. *The Psychology of Childbirth*. Cambridge, MA: Harvard University Press, 1978.

McBride, A. "Compulsory Rooming-in in the Ward and Private Newborn Service at Duke Hospital." *Journal of the American Medical Association*, vol. 145 (1951).

McKay, Susan, and Celeste R. Phillips. *Family Centered Maternity Care*. Rockville, MD: Aspen Systems Corporation, 1984.

Mehl, L. "Research on Alternatives: What It Tells Us About Hospitals." In Stewart, D., and L. Stewart, eds., *21st Century Obstetrics Now*, vol. 1. Marble Hill, MO: NAPSAC International.

Mehl, Lewis, et al. "Evaluation of outcomes of non-nurse midwives: Matched comparisons with physicians." *Women and Health*, vol. 5 (1980).

Midwives' Chronicle and Nursing Notes (July 1989).

Minkoff, H., and R. Schwartz. "The Rising Cesarean Section Rate: Can It Safely Be Reversed?" *Obstetrics and Gynecology*, vol. 4, no. 2 (August 1980).

Montgomery, T. "A Case for Nurse-Midwives." *American Journal of Obstetrics and Gynecology*, vol. 109.

National Institutes of Health. *Antenatal Diagnostics*, pub. no. 79-1973 (April 1979), Bethesda, MD.

Newton, Niles. "The Effect of Fear and Disturbance in Labor." *21st Century Obstetrics Now*, Stewart & Stewart, eds. Marble Hill, MO: NAPSAC Publications, 1977.

_____. *Maternal Emotions*. New York: Paul B. Hoeber, 1982.

Nurse-Midwifery in America, ed. Judith Rooks, CNM, and Eugene Haas, PhD. American College of Nurse-Midwives.

Odent, Michel. *Birth Reborn*. New York: Random House, 1984.

Oski, F. A. "Oxytocin and Hyperbilirubinemia." *American Journal of Dis. Child*, vol. 129 (1975).

Ostrowsky, L. L. *Alternative Birth Centers*. Berkeley, CA: Department of Health Services, 1982.

Paul, R.; J. Huey; and C. Yeager. "Clinical Fetal Monitoring: Its Effect on Cesarean Section Rate and Perinatal Mortality: Five-Year Trends." *Postgraduate Medicine*, vol. 61 (1977).

Peterson, G. Unpublished manuscript cited in *21st Century Obstetrics Now*. Marble Hill, MO: NAPSAC Publications, 1977.

Reinke, Carla. "Outcomes of the First 527 Births at The Birthplace in Seattle." *Birth*, vol. 9, no. 4 (1982).

Roberts, Joyce. "Alternative positions for childbirth, Part I: First stage of labor," and "Part II: Second stage of labor." *Journal of Nurse-Midwifery*, vol. 25 (1980).

Rosenthal, Michael. 1988. *Pre- and Perinatal Psychology News*, vol. II, issue I.

Russell, J. "The Rationale of Primitive Delivery Positions." *British Journal of Obstetrics and Gynecology*, vol. 89 (1982).

Sagov, Stanley, et al. *Home Birth: A Practitioner's Guide to Birth Outside the Hospital*. Rockland, MD: Aspen Systems Corp., 1984.

Sculphome, A.; A. G. McLeod; and E. G. Robertson. "A Birth Center Affiliated with the Tertiary Care Center: Comparison of Outcome." *Obstetrics and Gynecology*, vol. 67, no. 4 (April 1986).

Searles, Carolyn. "The impetus toward home birth." *Journal of Nurse-Midwifery*, vol. 26 (1985).

Shy, Kirkwood K., et al. "Effects of Electronic Fetal-Heart-Rate Monitoring as Compared with Periodic Auscultation on the Neurologic Development of Premature Infants." *New England Journal of Medicine*, March 1, 1990.

Shy, Kirkwood; Floyd Frost; and Jean Ullom. "Out-of-hospital delivery in Washington State, 1975–77." *American Journal of Obstetrics and Gynecology*, vol. 137 (1980).

Sidenbladh, Eric. *Water Babies*. New York: St. Martin's Press, 1982.

Stewart, David, PhD. "The Five Standards of Safe Childbearing." Marble Hill, MO: NAPSAC Publications, 1981.

Sullivan, Deborah A., and Rose Weitz. *Labor Pains: Modern Midwives and Home Birth*. New Haven, CT: Yale University Press, 1988.

Varney, Helen. *Nurse-Midwifery*. Boston: Blackwell Scientific Publications, 1980.

Wagner, G. Marsden. "Infant Mortality in Europe: Implications for the United States." *Journal of Pubic Health Policy*, Winter 1988.

Wertz, Richard W., and Dorothy C. Wertz. *A History of Childbirth in American*. New York: Schocken Books, 1979.

Williams, J. Kell, M.D. and Mathew R. Mervis, M.D. "Use of the labor-delivery-recovery room in an urban care hospital." *American Journal of Obstetrics and Gynecology*, vol. 162 (1990).